Badass
Advocate

Becoming the Champion Your Seriously Ill
Loved One Deserves

Erin Mulqueen Galyean

Cover creation: Deividas Jablonskis
Editing: Elizabeth Stockton
Formatting: Debbie Lum

ISBN: 978-1-7343460-0-8

Download a *FREE* copy of the
Badass Advocate
Action Guide

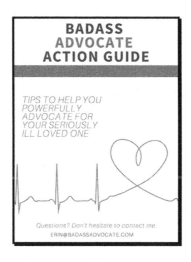

As a thank you for buying my book,
I would like to offer you a **free** *copy of the*
Badass Advocate Action Guide.

To download your free action guide, go to:
www.badassadvocate.com/actionguide

To my sister, Meghan,

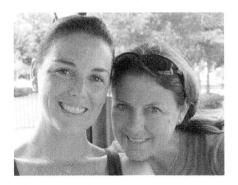

who showed us all what it meant to be truly selfless.

To my father, Mike,

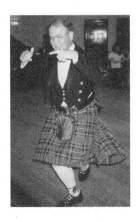

who taught us the importance of laughing your way through life.

I miss you both every day.

Table of Contents

Foreword
By Dr. Jennifer Aron

It was the spring of 2018, and I was working on an inpatient palliative care consult service. I'm a palliative care physician. My focus is to care for patients and their families suffering from life-limiting diseases. These patients need help with symptom management, extra support, advance care planning, goals of care discussions, and often some combination of the above.

On this day, the patient I was asked to see was a young woman in the Intensive Care Unit with respiratory failure from a severe lung disease that developed as a consequence of her cancer. She was a mother of young children, a wife, a daughter, a sister.

I clearly remember walking into the patient's room. Her name was Meghan, and I was warmly greeted by the patient, her sister, and her mother. In that first meeting I remember notepads and pens, lists of questions, but most importantly, strength and love.

That is how I first met the author, Erin Galyean. She was Meghan's sister.

Meghan was quite ill by the time I met her. What was obvious to me early in our relationship, in addition to Meghan's determination, was the dedication of the advocates that Meghan had in her corner. They were organized, proactive, and committed to not only ensuring Meghan received the best possible care, but also that she felt loved and supported through every turn.

They did not hide from difficult conversations, and they worked collaboratively with the healthcare team. They deferred to Meghan primarily, but when she was unable to process information herself, they advocated on her behalf. They supported Meghan and one another to navigate a truly heart-wrenching reality.

Meghan remains close to my heart still. She described herself once to me as a warrior, and that is how I remember her. I believe she was helped to stay a warrior until her last breath because of the advocacy of those who surrounded and loved her until the end.

The reality of a life-threatening illness is that there's no easy road through it. Families find themselves with the rug pulled from underneath them, with the trajectory of their lives forever changed.

To navigate the path requires collaboration and communication between patients, families, physicians, nurses, pharmacists, and insurance companies, just to name a few. It can be a daunting task, especially for the patient who is sick and the family who is reeling.

The caregiver often takes on the role of patient advocate, be that a spouse, a parent, a child, a close friend, or a team of all of the above. Having an advocate to help coordinate care, hear information and ask questions, organize transportation, manage medications, and—most importantly—provide support can be indispensable. A support team does not have to be large to be successful, and having a guidebook to help navigate this new, foreign terrain can be incredibly helpful.

In this book, Erin shares lessons learned from her own experiences as an advocate to help others jump into the role quickly and with a solid framework to build upon. I know personally that Erin and her family's ability to advocate for their loved one was impressive. Meghan's caregivers were able to support her and promote her goals and wishes to improve the quality of her care and the quality of her life.

The role of palliative care is also to act as an advocate for patients and families and to provide support during a difficult time. For families like Meghan's, we work alongside the support team already in place. For others who find themselves with less support or feel overwhelmed by the diagnosis, the medical jargon, the appointments, and the decisions, we are there to help provide some solid ground in the midst of quicksand.

If you or a loved one find yourself with a life-limiting illness, know that we are out there to help strengthen your voice. Please seek us out. Along with resources like this book, we can help provide a higher quality of care.

For some of you reading this book, there will be a happy ending to your journey. For others, you will face the unimaginable. But as I witnessed with Meghan and her family and friends, there are so many gifts to be shared, so many joys to be enjoyed, and so much life to be lived—even in the midst of critical illness and even in the face of death. I hope you can find those moments, and I wish you love and healing as you move forward.

"A happy life consists not in the absence but in the mastery of hardships."

~ *Helen Keller*

Contracted a childhood illness that left her blind and deaf

My Story

DAD

I was 19 years old when my father was diagnosed with non-Hodgkin's lymphoma (NHL). It was the summer of 1996, and it was an exciting new season of my life. I had just transferred to the University of North Carolina Chapel Hill.

I was thrilled to be at a larger, more prestigious school with a well-known sports program. I was eager for a fresh start and to make new friends.

It was a few weeks into the school year, and everything seemed to be going smoothly. I was navigating the new campus, bonding with my suitemates, and enjoying challenging classes. I was living the life of an average college student, worried about grades but focused on my social life.

That is, until I received a phone call from my parents. I answered the phone, and both of my parents were on the other line, which was unusual. I figured they were checking in on me since I was at a new school.

The conversation started out normal. They asked me about my new roommate and classes. Then the conversation took a sharp turn. That is when they tag-teamed in explaining what had transpired since I left home.

The short version is that my father had gone to the doctor for back pain, which he had dealt with for years. After additional testing they discovered that he had cancer, non-Hodgkin's lymphoma. Their tones sounded positive for the most part. I could sense they were trying to downplay the scariness of the situation. They did their best to convince me that he was going to be okay.

Regardless of what they said, I was scared, overwhelmed, and in disbelief.

As tears fell from my cheeks, I frantically blurted out, "I want to come home. I can transfer to a local school, live at home, and help with Dad."

They must have anticipated that this would be my response. Their answer was quick and final, "That is out of the question."

My dad particularly insisted that I stay in school. After all, getting into UNC Chapel Hill was a big accomplishment. Although I worked hard at getting good grades, I wasn't exactly a straight-A student. My entire family was so excited and proud when I was accepted. They didn't want me to give up this great opportunity. So, even though my heart was pulling me home, I stayed in North Carolina.

COMING HOME

I did come back home to Philadelphia when I could. But, this wasn't very often due to the distance between it and Chapel Hill.

When any of us kids came home, we habitually entered the house through the garage. My first visit home after Dad's chemo treatments, I did the same. But this time, I stopped for a moment to catch my breath. I needed to mentally prepare. I reassured myself that I could do this, that I could face my dad without crying.

Prior to coming home, I had been warned by my mom and sister that he looked drastically different. I was determined not to walk in the door, get one glance of him, and burst into tears. I suspected that doing so would break his heart.

So, I took a deep breath and braced myself. I gently opened the door and tiptoed into the kitchen. I found my sweet Dad exactly where I imagined him to be, resting in his leather chair.

They were right: he did look drastically different. He had completely transformed into an old man. Dad went from a strong, stout, and balding middle-aged man to a frail, small-boned, and hairless one.

He smelled different, too. Instead of the familiar smell of his aftershave that I came to recognize as his, he now smelled medicinal.

He awoke, we embraced, and I managed to hold back my tears until I got to my room. It was a severe change that was hard to accept. In the end, my family had no choice and it became our new norm.

The school year ended in May, and I returned home for the summer. To my dismay, less than two months after being home, my father would pass away. He died at the hospital, surrounded by our little family unit.

I was thankful that I was there, but at the same time, I was forever scarred by the memory of his passing. Because I had been at school since August, I didn't do much caretaking during his illness. Consequently, his death was quite shocking. Clearly, I knew he was sick. I just didn't realize the severity of his illness.

My parents had always stayed positive. They reassured my siblings and me that Dad was going to pull through. So, life carried on. I had no idea that before summer would end, he would be gone.

Meghan

Fast-forward 21 years, and we were doing well as a family. We each went through a grieving process in our own way.

We never would stop missing our dad. He was a big, bright light in our family. He always made everything seem fun and light-hearted. However, we were managing to cope with our loss.

We talked about him regularly. Since he had such a great sense of humor, the funny stories were endless. We enjoyed reminiscing about our crazy family adventures. Often, we would do our best to retell Dad's favorite jokes. These things seemed to help with the grieving process.

At this time, my brother (Michael), sister (Meghan), and I were all married. We each had children of our own. We were successful in our own right and living generally happy lives. Then, September 13, 2017 came, and once again we received life-altering news.

As a corporate sales trainer, I work from home, and that day, as I sometimes do, I decided to work at a local coffee shop. I remember my husband calling and asking me where I was working, which was unusual. Once I gave him the name of the coffee shop, he quickly replied that he was close by. He casually asked if I could come outside to see him. My birthday was just around the corner, so I got excited, thinking he was surprising me with lunch or a gift. Boy, was I sorely mistaken.

After I jumped into the car, I immediately recognized that something was wrong. His serious facial expression indicated I may not be getting a fun birthday surprise.

I deliberately turned to face him as he stumbled over his words. He searched for a way to inform me of the bad news. My sister had NHL— the same cancer my dad had.

My stomach dropped as I realized my biggest fear had become a reality. This could not be happening. Again.

Disorganized thoughts began taking over my mind. I frantically replayed scenes from the past 5 months. Repeating conversations I'd had with my sister, my heart began to race.

"No, this can't be true," I begged. "Please, this can't happen again."

I immediately burst into tears and sobbed uncontrollably. My husband rubbed my back consoling me, "I know. I'm so sorry, babe."

Meghan and I were born six years apart, but those years didn't prevent us from building a tight bond. Her personality was like my father's— kind, loving, and caring.

In 43 years, we got into two fights. That's not a typo. Only two. I admit both times I was being the bratty little sister. Although she had the patience of a saint, she wasn't going to take my crap.

If she wasn't so easy-going, then those two fights would have probably been more like 52. I was lucky to have been born her sister, and I always knew it. I'm thankful to say it wasn't something I ever took for granted.

THE DIAGNOSIS

I was so confused as to how she could contract the same cancer that our father had. We had always been told NHL wasn't genetic. The fact that Meghan had the same cancer as my dad was purely coincidental.

Furthermore, my sister was also a relatively healthy adult. She had been a Division-1 collegiate athlete and never smoked a cigarette or done drugs in her life. She worked out regularly and prided herself on eating a healthy diet.

Out of all people, how could this happen to her? Why did it have to happen to her? These were questions to which we would never get answers.

What I also didn't know that day was that the diagnosis of NHL was the good news. It was the curable type. At the time, I wasn't even aware that there were different types of NHL.

According to her physicians, "If you are going to get NHL, this is the strand you want." So, we relaxed. We took a collective deep breath and knew we'd help her fight through the cancer. She was a fighter, so we were confident she could get through this.

A Bomb Drops

Six months prior to her cancer diagnosis, Meghan was diagnosed with an autoimmune disease called Oral Lichen Planus (OLP). OLP causes the patient to have sores, and hers showed up in her mouth. It was an awful experience for her. Subsequently, she began losing weight rapidly since eating was so painful.

Now we knew she had two diseases, OLP and NHL, but what came next was the biggest shock.

When she was first diagnosed with NHL, Meghan went to the emergency room because she was having difficulty breathing. After her diagnosis, she stayed the night for further examination. Unfortunately, the doctors couldn't identify the cause of her breathing issues. They didn't think it was the cancer that was causing it. After a few days and many tests later, she was finally diagnosed with Bronchiolitis Obliterans (BO).

BO, also known as "popcorn lung," is an aggressive lung disease. What happens is the tiny air passages in your lungs begin to scar. The scarring causes a blockage that makes breathing difficult. As the disease progresses, the patient's breathing becomes severely labored.

You may recall from biology class that we breathe in oxygen and breathe out carbon dioxide (CO_2). Since BO causes the small air passages in the lungs to constrict, the CO_2 gets trapped. Trapped CO_2 then poisons the patient from the inside. It's horrifying.

Meghan's doctors concluded that the cancer caused the autoimmune disease. Then, the autoimmune disease caused the lung disease. For 13 months, we frantically searched for answers. In the end, answers wouldn't matter.

RAPID DECLINE

Meghan's doctors agreed that she had to tackle the cancer *before* they could address the lung disease. The challenge was that some of the lung disease medications couldn't be taken in conjunction with her chemotherapy drugs.

Like an athlete facing their toughest opponent, Meghan announced that she was going to "kick cancer's ass." As usual, she had a positive outlook.

Like many cancer patients, Meghan lost weight and hair early on. Her energy levels sharply declined, and she had little appetite. But what made fighting the cancer even more challenging was dealing with a lung disease at the same time.

By the start of 2018, it was obvious her breathing had worsened. Immediately following her diagnosis in September of 2017, she only needed an oxygen machine at night while she slept. But by January, she needed the oxygen during the day to help her get around. She was becoming more dependent on the oxygen machine, which wasn't a good sign. Understandably, this was also taking a toll on her emotionally and mentally.

Meghan's rapid decline was disheartening. Her lung disease had clearly worsened—its aggressiveness was frightening. Her doctors had warned us that, as the lung disease progressed, the damage couldn't be reversed. And she wouldn't be able to qualify for a lung transplant until she was cancer free for three or four years. At this pace, we weren't sure if she would even last a year.

Nevertheless, we stayed in fight mode. We remained hopeful that once her chemo treatments were over, the pulmonology team could stop the lung disease from advancing. We knew her lifestyle would drastically change, but we hoped that she could still live a long life.

In February, Meghan finished her chemo treatments. A few weeks later, we were told that she was cancer free. We were desperate for good news, and finally we got some. We were thrilled. She did kick cancer's ass. At last, we could focus on her lung disease.

As spring turned into summer, Meghan's lung disease continued to be managed through breathing treatments, medications, and physical therapy. Unfortunately, the many side effects of her lung disease caused her to spend a lot of time in and out of the hospital. Multiple times, she was rushed to the hospital due to labored breathing or an elevated heart rate.

When this happened, she would spend several days in the ICU as the staff worked to get her CO_2 levels, heart rate, and breathing under control. Once that was accomplished, she would move to the hospital's general ward. Eventually, she would be discharged. This process took weeks. Even worse, each hospital visit seemed to set her further back.

Over a short 13-month period, we watched as Meghan went from a vibrant, active, and independent woman into an easily fatigued, frail, and dependent patient. It was painful and heartbreaking to watch Meghan's body deteriorate. No matter what the doctors did for her, the lung disease intensified.

In the end, Meghan's body succumbed to her lung disease on October 13, 2018. She died three days shy of her 48th birthday.

TRYING MY BEST

Throughout her illness, I continued to travel back and forth from Texas to South Carolina. It wasn't easy, considering I had a young family of my own, but I was determined to be an influential advocate. Meghan was my lifelong best friend. Although I was living hundreds of miles away, I wasn't going to let distance prevent me from supporting her. My plan was to keep advocating for her until she was done fighting.

I had lingering regrets of not being a better advocate for my dad during his illness. Sure, I was young, naïve, and away at college during my father's illness. But understanding that doesn't change the regrets you can feel after you lose a person you love so much. I was not about to make the same mistake with Meghan.

As her condition worsened, it was clear that my skills and experience as a pharmaceutical sales trainer were a real asset when advocating. My knowledge gave me a different perspective and helped me to be an effective and capable patient advocate. My family went through such difficult experiences with both Meghan and my dad, but we also learned some valuable lessons about patient care and coordination. I didn't want those lessons to go to waste, and I became motivated to share them with others. That's why I created the Badass Advocate program—so readers, like you, can quickly become a Badass Advocate for the ones they love.

Now that you understand why my past has led me to write this book, let me share with you what I learned.

"Being challenged in life is inevitable, being defeated is optional."

~ Roger Crawford

The first person to play Division-1 tennis and work as a US tennis pro with a severe disability

Introduction
You Are Not Alone

Suddenly, you have found yourself in the most dreaded situation. Someone near and dear to your heart has become seriously ill. You desperately want to help, but you aren't exactly sure where to start.

You aren't a healthcare professional. You don't have a medical degree. You are overwhelmed by the barrage of information from the physicians and nurses. You aren't sure of what to ask or which direction to take.

You are caught in a vortex of wondering why your loved one drew the short stick. You ask yourself, *"How will I manage to get through it and when will I escape this newfound hell?"* In a nutshell, you feel lost, overwhelmed, and powerless.

If any of this sounds familiar, this book is for you.

This book will return a feeling of control and serve as a guide on how to be a Badass Advocate for your loved one. Here is how I define "Badass Advocate":

> *A Badass Advocate intentionally takes a strategic approach to caregiving. They are willing to step out of their comfort zone and go above and beyond to serve the patient. They act respectfully while acting on the behalf of the patient. They are determined, persistent, and empathetic. They create a healthy balance of taking care of the patient while also taking care of themselves.*

You might be reading this now, thinking, 'That's how I want to act. But I'm tired, confused, and unsure how to move forward.' Don't worry. That's exactly what this book will teach you. I'll take you through eight steps you can follow—starting today—to transform you into a Badass Advocate.

You can think of this book as your handbook to becoming a Badass Advocate. Everyone's situation is very personal, so take from it what will help. I don't expect you to implement every little idea I recommend. Rather, take the ideas that speak to you most and will work for your situation.

Keep this book handy to help build a strong sense of what it means to be a Badass Advocate. As a caretaker, you need to feel empowered. You need to believe that you can make a meaningful difference in your loved one's healthcare experience. Know that you *can* make an impact, and this book will help you get there.

I GET IT

Please know that I empathize with what you are going through. I've lost two out of my four immediate family members to aggressive diseases. One I lost to cancer; the other to a lung disease. Both had a strong will to live and a positive outlook, but unfortunately, both died way too young.

My father died at age 53 and my sister at 47. They both spent a significant amount of time in and out of the hospital. They also didn't live long after their diagnoses. This was disheartening and shocking to all who loved them.

Having a seriously ill loved one is a torturous and emotional rollercoaster ride. It can be a constant cycle of worry and then relief, worry and then relief. I know all too well this horrible feeling of helplessness.

My mission is to turn my personal story into something positive. I know my story is like many others, but at the same time, each person's journey is unique. In sharing what I've learned, I hope you will become a Badass Advocate yourself.

Throughout this book, I'll share stories of how my family advocated for my sister. I'll tell you how you can put these ideas into practice so that your loved one can get the care they deserve. In fact, you'll have an advantage over me: you'll be going in with a plan.

First, you'll learn how to create a strong and powerful army of advocates. Then, you'll learn techniques to help that army better work *with* healthcare providers. Next, we will focus on how to take better care of yourself and the patient. Last, you will learn how to put these tips to use. Each tip is practical and actionable, leaving you in more control in a turbulent time.

My Personal Experience

On top of my personal trauma, I have over 19 years of experience in the pharmaceutical sales industry. Throughout my career, I've trained salespeople how to better communicate with others. This includes physicians, co-workers, and executives. This knowledge was an asset to me when advocating for my sister. In this book, I'll share some of those strategies with you.

One such example (Badass Strategy #4) is recording conversations with the patient and the physician. This practice allowed us to better understand what was going on with our sick loved one. After recording conversations, we could confidently share information with absent family members. This practice aligned and strengthened our support team. Recording conversations was one of many great ideas we put into practice.

Another useful tip is Badass Strategy #8: a daily routine that will help you easily put all the Badass Strategies into practice. My hope is that this routine will help minimize your stress, keep you focused, and enable you to start your day off strong. Because regardless of your situation, every Badass Strategy will lead you to becoming a Badass Advocate.

IMPORTANCE OF ADVOCATING

After each chapter, I've included a list of Badass Advocate Actions. These are specific, actionable items that you can use immediately. I encourage you to implement as many of these actions as possible. Don't be the person who waits and then regrets not taking steps that could have made a difference in your loved one's care. You need to start advocating *today*. The sooner you can be their champion, the bigger difference you can make in their care.

Let me give you an example of why patient advocacy is so important, even when the patient you are advocating for is yourself.

While I was writing this book, my best friend of 20 years was diagnosed with cancer. She is 48 years old, and this is her third cancer diagnosis—two times with breast cancer and now with endometrial cancer.

Before her diagnosis, she had been experiencing some odd symptoms. Intuition told her something with her body was off. So, she booked appointments with different specialists. Yet, each appointment left her with no answers and more questions.

Due to the breast cancer, she had been taking a drug to manage her estrogen. With this drug came a small risk of causing endometrial cancer. Yet, as she pursued answers for her mysterious symptoms, not one physician mentioned endometrial cancer as a possibility. Instead, each physician came up with a different theory, none of which ended up being correct.

To be fair, the risk of this drug causing endometrial cancer is quite low; it occurs in only 1% of patients taking the drug. Yet, the risk remains, and her doctors did not investigate it.

She ultimately found out she had endometrial cancer because *she* acted as her own advocate. When she wasn't getting the answers she needed, she didn't give up. She didn't throw in the towel and think, "I'll just deal with these symptoms." She followed her gut and kept fighting for herself.

As a result, she found a physician who did the right testing and uncovered the endometrial cancer. Thankfully, endometrial cancer is slow growing, so her prognosis is a positive one. But if left untreated, it can spread.

I share her story because I want to strongly impress upon you the importance of patient advocacy. In this case, the patient was healthy enough that she could advocate for herself. But often patients facing these kinds of diagnoses are not strong enough to advocate for themselves. They need someone else to step in and be the Badass Advocate that everyone deserves.

Being a vocal advocate does not mean being an antagonist to medical professionals. It is important to recognize that physicians are humans, and they can make mistakes. Many of our diseases are still a mystery, and physicians sometimes simply do not yet have all the answers. Therefore, you need to be diligent, vocal, and strong for the patient.

Throughout this journey, you will need to fight for your loved one to get them the care they need. When I say "fight," I do not mean go to battle with medical professionals. These professionals have many patients to care for and many responsibilities. Your job is to pay close attention to *your* loved one's case and make sure nothing is overlooked. Get the answers you need so they can get the care they desire.

Also, I must point out that before you undertake any action, you need to consult the patient first. You should never make decisions about someone else's healthcare on your own. If the patient is alert and coherent, then they need to be in charge. It is their health and their body, and your job is to support them.

I wish you and your sick loved one the best through this challenging journey. I hope that reading this book will help you to realize you aren't alone. Many people have gone through such challenging times. Some people may be quiet about these experiences, but they are out there, dealing with the same kind of heartache.

I also want to say to you that I am truly sorry. I am sorry you are experiencing this level of fear, pain, and sadness. I am sorry you must watch your loved one suffer. No matter your situation, it's awful, and I'm sorry you must go through it.

Last, I am confident you can make a difference in your loved one's care. It may not be easy. Some days you will be exhausted. But your actions do matter. To that I say, soldier on, my friend. You got this. And I'm here to help.

Let's make you a badass.

"Unity is strength…when there is teamwork and collaboration, wonderful things can be achieved."

~ Mattie Stepanek

Before dying at age 13 from a rare form of muscular dystrophy, Mattie was a poet, advocate, and motivational speaker

Badass Strategy #1
Build a Support Team

In this chapter, I'll explain why good teamwork is fundamental for becoming a Badass Advocate. I'll give you suggestions on how to select your team members, what roles they can play, and how you can foster successful teamwork. This will enable you to create a strong team of advocates right away.

WHY A SUPPORT TEAM

The first step I recommend is to prepare for the battle ahead. You prepare by building a support team—a small army of people who will commit to making sacrifices to support the patient. There are two main reasons why building an official support team is crucial:

1. If a patient is seriously ill, they cannot possibly manage their own care. The patient's main job is to focus on getting well. That is why they need loyal individuals to fight for them. They will need support on days when they're feeling weak, their mind is fuzzy, or they don't have the energy to talk. These days can come and go.

2. Caregiving often naturally falls on one person's shoulders, such as a spouse or parent. This is why a support team is critical. When it comes to patient caregiving, there is a great deal of responsibility. The job is simply is too much for one individual

to handle. Being a caretaker can also be a thankless job, so it's important to have a team of partners to support you.

If you are struggling to think of who can join the support team, keep reading. You may not have a large group of family members to choose from, and that is okay. You can still build a support team with friends.

Remember, having a team of caregivers will help balance out responsibilities. If you can delegate even minor tasks, it will help.

BUILDING A SUPPORT TEAM

If you can assemble an army of advocates from the start, you will be ahead of the game. For example, you may have many family members who live nearby. If this is the case for you, then building a support team may be a no-brainer. But, I realize not everyone has this luxury. If you do not have a team of helpful family members nearby, you will need to depend on loyal and reliable friends and members of the community. Regardless, you need to start building your army immediately.

I encourage you to read through this chapter first, and then begin to reach out for help. Being a one-person support team is terribly difficult. And if you want to be a Badass Advocate, then assembling an army of advocates should be your first step.

CHOOSING MEMBERS

There will be people who will naturally be part of the patient's army, like their spouse or their adult child, and others may not be so obvious. But it's important to keep in mind that support team members will be around the patient *a lot*. Meaning, team members must be people whom the patient can tolerate and be comfortable around—especially when the patient is having a bad day.

When people get seriously ill, there may be times when they reach a new low that they never imagined. For example, they may lose control of their bowels, expose private parts, or exhibit strange behavior. Because of this, you'll need to verify that the patient won't be embarrassed if the people on your list are present.

As you begin to compile your list of candidates, consider the attributes listed below. Keep in mind: each member doesn't have to possess all the characteristics listed. But the more you can check off, the more success you will have in building a team of powerful advocates. If the scenario arises that one candidate doesn't have any of these attributes, then I recommend passing over that person.

TRUSTWORTHY

Support team members will hear sensitive health information. This means certain people, like the "town gossip," will not make a good advocate. All support team members need to respect the patient's privacy. They will need to have common sense as well as restraint. They need to understand that they are not permitted to share certain information with others.

EMOTIONALLY INTELLIGENT

Support team members are the eyes, ears, and memory of the patient. This happens because many patients are in shock when they receive upsetting news.

The harsh reality is that a healthcare provider could relay difficult news at any time and in any meeting. There is no way to mentally prepare for it. This means team members need to stay in tune with the patient and be prepared to act on their behalf.

One way team members can act on the patient's behalf is by continually asking questions. The goal should be to clearly understand the current situation, as well as what the next steps might be. I will give you some tips in Chapter 3 on effective questions to ask healthcare providers.

Also, your army needs to have enough emotional intelligence to understand social cues. The last kind of team member you want is one who irritates every healthcare professional they encounter.

RELIABLE

Seriously ill patients cannot afford to miss doctor's appointments. In other words, those responsible for taking the patient to appointments need to be reliable.

If the patient is hospitalized, at least one team member should be present when the hospitalists are making rounds. It's important to understand that rounds are an opportune time to gain information, ask questions, and understand the patient's status. I'll explain this more in-depth later.

Team members need to be reliable when it's their turn to be "on call."

PUNCTUAL

Reliability and punctuality are closely related attributes. But they are both so important I wanted to dive into each separately.

There will be occasions when a team member's presence will be required. For example, they may need to administer time-sensitive medication or accept a medical-related delivery. It is forgivable to be late from time to time, but habitual lateness can be detrimental to a patient's health. Plus, it can cause stress for everyone involved.

Anyone who needs to be on time for things like appointments needs to be punctual. If a team member has a reputation for being late, then assign them a role where punctuality is not as important. I will discuss these roles more in-depth in the Bonus section, so keep this one in mind.

EMOTIONALLY STRONG

No pun intended, but this trait is a tough one. When a loved one is sick, it can be challenging to be emotionally strong for them.

When out of sight of the patient, releasing your emotions is to be expected—and is also necessary. You may need to cry, scream, or vent. Go ahead and release your emotions. This is a difficult time and holding things in will only make it harder on you.

Yet, when in front of the patient, aim to be empathetic, but positive. Constantly showing your fear, sadness, or worry will not help the mental state of the patient. You want to support them and encourage them to think positively.

In "The Power of Positive Thinking,"[1] Johns Hopkins claims that a patient's positive mindset "improves outcomes and life satisfaction across a spectrum of conditions—including traumatic brain injury, stroke, and brain tumors." You may not be able to control the patient's attitude, but you can control your own. Furthermore, being surrounded by positive advocates can certainly influence the patient's outlook.

---

[1] https://www.hopkinsmedicine.org/health/wellness-and-prevention/the-power-of-positive-thinking

People who have the ability to be a bright light during a frustrating, scary, and dark time can be a huge benefit. Again, put yourself in the shoes of the patient. If you are having a rough day, would you rather be around someone who can lift your spirits or someone who is a Debbie Downer?

An easy way to lighten anyone's day is to smile. When my sister was sick, I had a lot of anxiety, so on many days I had to force myself to smile at her. Ultimately, I realized it not only helped to lighten her mood, but it helped my attitude as well.

My point is to be aware of your behavior in front of the patient, so you don't bring them down even further. If your goal is to be a Badass Advocate, then you must support the patient in having a positive mindset.

CONFIDENT

It's important that team members see themselves as working *with* the healthcare providers to do what's best for the patient. It's critical that they are eager and confident enough to speak to healthcare providers. Remember, advocates represent the patient.

Furthermore, there may be times when you need to "challenge" the healthcare provider. Team members need to be self-assured when these kinds of situations arise.

AVAILABLE

Availability may seem obvious, but it's important to think through. When I say "availability," I'm referring to both distance and accessibility.

The more local support the patient has, the better. Team members who live close by can be available for doctors' appointments, hospital visits, home health support, and more. They also can be called upon at a moment's notice for emergencies. Illness doesn't follow a schedule, and when someone is sick, they may need to be suddenly rushed to the hospital.

Availability during the week is also important if daily care is necessary. Most of your core team members may work, so finding weekday support may be a struggle. Do your best to add at least one person to the support team who can be available during the workweek. Finding someone local who is retired, is unemployed, or works from home may be a good fit.

Realize that team members who live long distance can still be a big asset. I will share how long-distance team members can help in the book. The overarching idea is to build a bench of local folks who are willing to do the heavy lifting. At the same time, use long-distance folks for tasks that can be accomplished via phone, text, or email.

ASK FOR HELP

In the end, don't be shy. Asking people to give so much may be uncomfortable. However, most people want to help, but they don't know how. Having them join the support team will enable them to meaningfully contribute.

If asking for help is challenging for you, remind yourself that this is what it takes to be a Badass Advocate. You are assembling a small army of advocates on behalf of the person you love. Yours is a noble cause.

If you come from a large family, review the list of characteristics and narrow down your team. The goal is to ensure there aren't too many people involved. Believe it or not, too many team members can create significant challenges, such as personality clashes and conflicting opinions. At some point, this situation may be a life-or-death one, so choose your team members wisely and try not to worry about hurting feelings.

If you are struggling to come up with support team members, below are some ideas for who you could consider:

- Spouse

- Siblings

- Parents (either patient's parents or spouse's parents)

- Friends (old and new)

- Cousins

- Aunts/Uncles

- Church members/clergyman

- Co-workers

- Neighbors

The point is you shouldn't go it alone. You will need to find others to help you even if it's just one person that can help with the smaller, less invasive tasks. For more ideas on how to delegate tasks, check out the Bonus section at the end of the book.

NUMBER OF MEMBERS

To give you an idea of how it worked for my family, my sister's support team consisted of about 10 people. About half were part of the core team, and the rest stepped in when extra support was needed. The extra support was critical for when core team members felt burnt out.

Once you have your support team in place, it's important to keep the group connected. You'll want everyone on the same page so that everything runs smoothly. Tips on how to make this happen will be covered in the Bonus section.

TEAM MEMBER ROLES

Below is a list of potential roles for your team. Certainly, you do not need to fill every role listed, but this list will give you a sense of what kind of services and organizational efforts may help your loved one. For smaller support teams, one person may need to own multiple roles. I provide detailed descriptions of each role in the Bonus section. The following is a brief overview:

Care Coordinator: This is the most important team member. This person manages, organizes, and coordinates the patient's care. To effectively manage the patient's care, buy a notebook dedicated to tracking the patient's key health information.

Support Team Leader: This person organizes, coordinates, and manages the support team. This team member assigns the roles to other team members and helps everyone stay connected.

Master of Medications: This team member learns about and manages the patient's medications.

Donations Manager: This person coordinates efforts to raise funds for the patient and their family.

Meal Train Organizer: This team member arranges, organizes, and manages meal donations.

Vice President of Communications: This person composes and sends messages about the patient's health and treatment to close family and friends. Having an open line of communication keeps non-support team members informed and notifies them of opportunities to support the patient.

Director of Delight: This team member focuses on lifting the patient's spirits, but also works to keep the entire team feeling supported and nurtured.

Before you jump into assembling your army, discuss the concept first with the patient. It's important to confirm that they agree with your plan. Remember this is their health journey, not yours. First, explain what a support team does for the patient and why it is important for both of you to rely on others. Then you can discuss what role each person will play.

When you discuss this idea with the patient, have a list of potential candidates on hand. Then, inform the patient that they are in charge and encourage them to give you feedback. Being in charge means they can veto your suggestions and add team members as needed.

During this conversation, try to avoid conflict. Stay focused on accomplishing the goal of building an army of advocates. This is a prime opportunity to encourage the patient to get the support they will need.

INVOLVE THE PATIENT

This leads me to one key principle you need to keep in mind while reading this book-always involve the patient. There is no doubt that as a

Badass Advocate you will be fighting hard for your loved one's health every chance you get. Your focus will be to get them the care they need to improve their experience. But while you are relentlessly supporting this person whom you love, there may be times when you unintentionally exclude them.

Forgetting to include the patient can happen more easily than you may think. After all, you are juggling a lot of balls. But regardless of all the distractions and responsibilities, you must prioritize the patient.

You will accomplish this by continually keeping them abreast of discussions about their care. Of course, this can be tricky for several very understandable reasons. Still, you should remind yourself that you are fighting for the health of *their* body.

> I vividly remember both my sister and my dad voicing concerns about being excluded from conversations about their care. Afterwards, they insisted that we include them.
>
> The incident I remember with my dad occurred while he was hospitalized. On this particular day, my mom was acting as my dad's advocate. She and the doctor were having a conversation about my dad's health a few feet away from his bed. Suddenly, he perked up and exclaimed, "Don't talk about me like I'm not here!" Both my mom and the doctor were shocked. This outburst was out of character for him.
>
> I am sure my mom and the doctor assumed my dad was sleeping and couldn't contribute to the conversation. At that time, he also had a tendency to have an unclear mind. Including him in every discussion wasn't always possible. Clearly, their intentions were virtuous. But, it is understandable why he became irritated and frustrated. He wanted to be the decision-maker.

My sister's frustrations stemmed more from the support team's behind-the-scenes work. I recall one time when our good intentions went awry. I was talking to Meghan about one of her physicians. I told her that I felt he "needed to be more proactive in his approach rather than reactive". To my surprise, she became irritated with me. I was caught off guard. Like my dad, this reaction was unusual.

Later I realized what happened. A few days earlier, I made the same comment to my mom when discussing Meghan's case. Our mom agreed a change needed to be made but that it wasn't up to her. It was my sister's decision. She was right.

As a good advocate would, our mom discussed this concern with my sister. While doing so, she used almost the exact same words I did. When I repeated those words a few days later, it clicked. At that point, Meghan realized that we were discussing her case when she wasn't present. From her perspective it felt we were conspiring behind her back.

In both incidences, it is easy to empathize with the patient. You can understand why our actions as support team members weren't well-received. To be fair, we had the best intentions and only wanted what was best for them. Yet, neither of them wanted to be treated like a child. They didn't appreciate being excluded from discussions about their own health.

This doesn't mean a fear of the patient feeling left out should prevent you from working on their behalf. Instead, the team should be cognizant of *prioritizing* the patient when advocating. A best practice is to inform the patient ahead of time of your plan. Inform them that in some incidences the team may need to have conversations without them. But then also reassure them that all conversations will be in their best interest.

Finally, the team needs to commit to always circling back with the patient. It is critical that the patient knows that they are the final decision maker. This practice may help your loved one feel in control and supported at the same time.

INCOHERENT PATIENTS

Even if the patient isn't responsive, you can still include them in the discussion. First, you will want to ask the patient one question at a time in a slow-paced manner. If the patient doesn't answer you, ask again a bit more forcefully. Ensure that what you are saying is simple and clear. If the patient still doesn't respond, inform them that you plan to go ahead. But, reassure them that you welcome their comments and input at any point.

This may sound something like:

> *"Mom, I'm going to talk with the doctor a bit about your medication. Is that ok? (no response) Mom, did you hear me? I'm going to talk to the doctor about your medication. Do you have anything you want to add or ask? (no response) Mom, if you decide you want to say something, we will be right here."*

If you think the person isn't listening or able to contribute, this is still a good practice. Badass Advocates must always try to get the patient's input when they can.

HEALTHCARE PROXY

If the patient is lucid and able to make their own health decisions, then legally no one can do it for them. The one exception is if the patient has given someone else that right. For example, an elderly patient may entrust an adult child to make medical decisions for them. In other words, they relinquish the decision-making even when they are coherent.

Then, there may be times when your loved one is so sick that they are incapable of making decisions on their own. For example, the patient may be in a coma, heavily medicated, or severely confused. If this happens they will need someone to make healthcare decisions for them.

Before the patient lacks this capacity, ask them to designate a healthcare proxy. A healthcare proxy is a person chosen by the patient to make healthcare decisions on their behalf. This is critical because if a patient becomes too ill, they will need someone else to step into this role. They should have the power to decide who this person will be.

If your loved one does not designate a healthcare proxy, then the medical staff will defer to the next of kin. The issue is that the next of kin may not be who the patient would want to make healthcare decisions on their behalf. As you can imagine, this situation can get quite complicated and sticky.

As a Badass Advocate, you should encourage your loved one to name a healthcare proxy. Knowing your loved one's exact wishes is essential. No one can anticipate what will happen to a seriously ill patient. Hopefully, the healthcare proxy will never be called upon. But if the patient takes a turn for the worse, you will be thankful to know who they want to be in control.

Advance Directive

To take it one step further, you should encourage your loved one to fill out an advance directive. An advance directive is a set of legal documents that define a patient's wishes regarding their end-of-life care. This may include documents like a living will, healthcare proxy, and healthcare power of attorney.

If you aren't sure where to begin, speak to your doctor, lawyer or hospital chaplain for help. Even for loved ones who are expected to recover, filling out an advance directive is a wise decision.

Support Tools

If you'd like advice on how to approach your loved one about advance care planning, check out the organization Aging with Dignity. Aging with Dignity is a non-profit organization whose mission is to help terminally ill patients die with dignity. On their website, they provide a document titled "The Conversation Guide for Individuals and Family". This guide helps advocates to better navigate this sometimes difficult and uncomfortable conversation. For a link to this document, you can go to www.badassadvocate.com/resources.

Aging with Dignity also provides a very helpful booklet called Five Wishes®. This booklet guides the patient in making five key critical health decisions. The first "wish" gives the patient direction on how to choose a healthcare proxy.

I'd like to point out a few key points about Five Wishes®. First, it is best if the patient answers the questions while they are coherent. Each "wish" is a major healthcare decision. Also, it's good to note that Five Wishes® replaces any directives the patient had in place before. You'll want to make sure the patient is aware of this change. Last, it is valid in only 42 states, so before relying on it, ensure it meets the legal requirements of your state.

Conclusion

The most important take away from this chapter—which I cannot stress enough—is to ask for help. Taking care of a seriously ill patient can be challenging, overwhelming, and stressful in so many ways. That is why asking for support is a must. Even if you only ask others to assume small, menial tasks, it can make a big difference.

Your goal as a Badass Advocate isn't to prove you can do it by yourself. Rather your focus should be on the patient and getting them the best care possible. Obtaining premium care will not be possible if you are burnt out.

Badass Advocate Actions:

- ☐ First, educate the patient on why building a support team is important to their health. Then, confirm they are onboard with the idea.

- ☐ Once the patient is aligned, discuss possible candidates. Consider the attributes mentioned in this chapter.

- ☐ Keep the team small enough so it is manageable and large enough that you have enough help. Even if you don't have a big support system, figure out ways to get others to help even if it's for taking over less important tasks.

- ☐ After checking off the above, start assembling your army. To build an army of Badass Advocates, only choose those who are willing to commit to supporting the patient long term.

- ☐ Involve the patient at every turn. Remember it is their health you are fighting for, not your own.

☐ Encourage the patient to fill out an advance directive, even if their prognosis is a positive one. Knowing what their end-of-life wishes are will only bring you comfort if the situation should arise.

♡

"A hero is an ordinary individual who finds the strength to persevere and endure in spite of overwhelming obstacles."

~ Christopher Reeve

After becoming a quadriplegic from being thrown from a horse, Reeve became an activist for people with disabilities & spinal cord injuries

Badass Strategy #2
Be Persistent and Respectful

Many of us hold physicians in high regard. For good reason, we respect their years of dedication and commitment to healing the sick. Our high regard for physicians isn't a bad thing unless it prevents us from being an effective advocate.

Some put physicians on such a high pedestal that they avoid any necessary pushback. People fear that questioning a doctor's decisions is insulting to the physician. They worry it may ruin the doctor/patient relationship. But voicing concerns *is* in the best interest of the patient. If you're not entirely comfortable with the idea of speaking up and maybe even pushing back to a team of medical professionals, then pay close attention to this chapter.

Badass Strategy #2 is about how to effectively give pushback while also being respectful. We will discuss why second opinions are important and when switching providers may be necessary. I will teach you a technique to help you remain calm, confident, and open-minded when challenging physicians. For those of you who get anxiety when confronting others, I recommend rereading this chapter when you anticipate facing one of these situations.

Do Your Research

If your gut tells you something is off, the first step you need to take is conducting your own research. Healthcare is a complex world, and new discoveries are found daily. This means there may be options the physician has not yet considered. Fighting for your loved one to get the best care requires that you research possible alternatives. In the end, you may discover that there aren't viable alternatives for you to pursue, but at the very least, it is worth looking into.

Start your research by collecting information from various reliable resources, including government websites, medical libraries, and other healthcare providers. Remember: anyone can post anything to the internet. Many websites may look legitimate but may contain misleading or anecdotal information. Keep this in mind before presenting opposing points of view to a doctor. Physicians can get frustrated when patients or their advocates bring inaccurate information forward based on their own Google searches.

On the other hand, many legitimate websites do provide valuable medical information. You just need to know where to find them. Reliable websites may offer published medical studies, articles, and books. Also, online libraries can help define medical jargon that may be foreign to you. Go to www.badassadvocate.com/resources for an updated list of reliable medical websites.

In reality, you will not always have time to conduct your own research before a critical conversation. If that is the case, asking questions is your best bet for gaining a clear understanding. Continue to ask questions respectfully until you are sure you understand what the physician is communicating. If possible, do research afterward and follow up later.

BE THEIR VOICE

Conducting research is only one step in advocating for better care. To be a Badass Advocate, you must be willing to be the patient's voice. Paying close attention and standing up for what is right are two important responsibilities that will most likely fall on your shoulders— especially if the patient doesn't have the energy or capability to do so for themselves. I'll warn you: doing this is not always an easy job.

As in any other profession, doctors have a range of personalities. Some doctors will be open to answering your concerns while others may cop an attitude. If you have been paying close attention and doing your research, be confident with your insights. Do not let a medical professional intimidate you. Stay focused on your goal of getting your loved one what they need.

You may not be a healthcare professional, but your thoughts are still important. For example, you know what the patient was like before they got sick, which is a valuable insight. The medical staff does not have this perspective. You, on the other hand, can recognize if a certain behavior is odd which may indicate if something is seriously wrong. Don't underestimate how important this perspective can be for a critical patient.

GETTING A SECOND OPINION

As someone who has seen two loved ones go through serious illnesses, I urge you to seek advice from at least one additional physician. This is especially important when you or the patient aren't getting answers to your concerns. Second opinions are important because physicians have widely varying experiences and research backgrounds. You never know when a doctor's knowledge may be the key to your loved one's recovery.

Seeking a second opinion may be uncomfortable. This is especially true if the patient has a strong relationship with their doctor. Having a strong bond with a physician usually equates to a high level of trust. That trust may have taken years to build and bring the patient the comfort they need.

On top of that, the patient doesn't want to insult their doctor who takes such good care of them. So, the patient may feel that asking for another physician's opinion is a betrayal. This is when changing your or the patient's mindset will help you to more powerfully advocate. I'd like you to think of getting a second opinion not as betraying the physician, but as fighting for the patient.

Each healthcare professional has different life experiences, professional knowledge, and medical community connections. Thus, one physician may treat the same disease differently than another. If there is even the slightest possibility that another doctor's insights can improve your loved one's health, then it is worth the effort.

Most physicians are making decisions to the best of their knowledge. However, if they are not an expert on this particular disease, then their knowledge may be limited. If the disease is rare, another physician may recommend a different treatment strategy.

If the physicians agree, even better. The second opinion will only build your confidence in what the first doctor told you. You will feel good knowing that the original physician is taking the right steps.

If you are still hesitant about asking for a second opinion, remind yourself that actively pursuing solutions is part of your responsibility as a Badass Advocate. Stay laser focused on the task at hand and proceed with determination to find answers.

Please know that the goal of seeking another doctor's opinion isn't to drag the patient around until someone gives you the answer you *want*. This is not what a Badass Advocate does. It is not in the best interest of the patient, and it will not improve their health.

If several physicians are giving you the same answers and the prognosis is not good, then rest assured you have your answer. I am sorry to say that you should then focus on accepting the situation for what it is and supporting the patient emotionally.

FINDING A SECOND OPINION

Finding someone to give you a second opinion is not necessarily a difficult task, but it may pose some challenges. For more common diseases, you should be able to find another specialist in your area. Keep in mind that doctors who are in high demand may not have an opening for a while. Depending on how dire the situation, this may pose an issue. Remember, the point of a second opinion is not to just get one, but to get one from someone who is an expert in the disease.

When finding experts on your loved one's disease, get creative. Ask family and friends for recommendations. They may have personal connections with experts who have the answers you need. This is why being open and sharing your news with others can be helpful.

Another way to seek a second opinion is through local charities that support your loved one's disease. A support team member can join the charity, attend events, and network within the community. People who join a charity are likely to be passionate about that disease and willing to help others. In fact, they may have experience with the same disease and have connections to an expert in this field.

If your loved one's disease is rare, getting a second opinion that is worthwhile may be more challenging. You may need to conduct in-depth research. The good news is you don't need to find someone locally to get a second opinion. You can conduct a nationwide search for physicians who are experts on your loved one's disease. Focus on those who are conducting current trials to see if you can benefit from their findings.

Once you discover a few experts, reach out via email or phone to explain your story and ask for help. If they offer their support, the patient can release their medical records. The new doctor can then review their case electronically. This is the beauty of technology.

The perspective of another physician can make a big difference in a patient's health. Let me share with you an example.

> If you've ever known a chemotherapy patient, you know how thin and frail they can become. On top of the chemo, Meghan's autoimmune disease caused her to have painful sores in her mouth. This made eating unappealing and caused rapid weight loss. Keeping weight on was almost impossible.
>
> At one point, Meghan weighed 86 pounds. It was horrifying.
>
> As you can imagine, the more weight she lost, the weaker she became. It's hard to fight a disease when you are exhausted and frail. We were beginning to realize that Meghan couldn't gain a pound on her own. Regardless of how many calorie-dense milkshakes she consumed, her weight declined. As it continued to drop, our concerns grew greater.
>
> That's when our Mom discussed the idea of a feeding tube with Meghan's pulmonary team. At the time, they felt it wasn't a good idea since a feeding tube could open her up to an infection. It was a risk they weren't willing to take.

This wasn't the answer we expected, but it seemed reasonable. After all, what did we know about feeding tubes? They were the professionals, right?

A few weeks later, a friend of my mom's emailed her a few articles and studies she found about Meghan's lung disease, Bronchiolitis Obliterans (BO). In her email she pointed out that one pediatric pulmonologist's name kept showing up. The doctor's name was Dr. Kirsten Williams. After reading what she had forwarded, it was clear that Dr. Williams was an expert on this rare disease.

I knew I had to reach out to Dr. Williams. If there was a small chance she could help, it was worth a shot. The worst thing that could happen was that she wouldn't respond.

To my surprise, not only did Dr. Williams respond, but she shared a great deal of valuable information. She wrote an empathetic note and attached an article that she had published on how to treat BO. She also offered to look at Meghan's chart, speak to her husband, and consult with Meghan's doctors, if we wanted. This was amazing!

Dr. Williams is one of those caring physicians who is generous with her time and knowledge. She didn't know my family, and we had no previous connection. But she was willing to go out of her way to help us.

She also gave us advice about what we could do for Meghan in the meantime. One of her top recommendations, *get her a feeding tube*. Dr. Williams explained that a BO patient's labored breathing will cause them to burn a lot of calories. Because of this, it makes gaining weight a real challenge. Therefore, if Meghan didn't get a feeding tube, she wouldn't gain weight. If she didn't gain weight, she couldn't build the strength to fight back.

Reread those last two sentences. Keep in mind: Meghan's pulmonology team told us she didn't need a feeding tube. This is exactly why I passionately voice the importance of doing research and seeking a second opinion.

In Meghan's case, the pulmonology team's hesitation to give her a feeding tube didn't make them bad physicians. They all had Meghan's best interest at heart. Dr. Williams just knew things about BO that her pulmonologists did not. Meghan's initial team saw the feeding tube issue one way, while Dr. Williams understood it differently. Based on her expertise, Dr. Williams knew the feeding tube was critical. Simple as that.

BE PERSISTENT

Being a Badass Advocate is not just about seeking a second opinion. Sometimes getting a second opinion will be as easy as booking an appointment. In other cases, it may become a real challenge. As a Badass Advocate, you need to have the courage to persistently follow up with those who are not responding.

If you don't get a response within a week, pursue one. Don't worry about being a pest. Naturally, you need to give the physician time to respond. Five to seven business days should be enough time. Embrace the Badass Advocate mindset. Be persistent!

If it brings you comfort, know that most physicians enter their profession because they want to help people. But they are also busy and may not spend much time in front of their computer. Your email might get lost in the shuffle, so don't hesitate to politely remind them of your request. Remember, seeking the advice of a few healthcare providers will give you balanced feedback and possibly new insights.

Now that you've done some research and obtained a second opinion, hopefully you agree with the first physician's plan of attack. If not, let's explore how to delicately and respectfully voice your concerns.

GIVING PUSHBACK (WHEN NECESSARY)

You have now armed yourself with knowledge. But knowledge is only powerful when you take action. As an advocate, you must share your concerns with the provider.

There is a four-step technique I teach sales reps to use when a physician has an opposing opinion. It can easily be applied to this situation. Let me share with you how you can use this technique to get your point across without causing tension.

1. *Acknowledge* the doctor's point of view. If you immediately begin disagreeing with the doctor's opinion, most likely you will cause them to get defensive. Reinforce that you believe they are trying to do what is best for the patient.

2. *Ask questions* to better understand why they feel this path is the best choice for your loved one. There may be reasonings you have not considered. Every patient is unique so get the answers to your specific concerns. Continue to ask questions until you are clear on why they've made certain decisions and recommendations.

3. *Explain* your perspective so the doctor understands why you have an opposing view. I highly recommend coming with alternative solutions based on what you have learned. If you

sought a second opinion and their plan was different, this is when you would share that information. Bring all relevant documentation to support why you disagree with the doctor's plan. Keep the discussion open by allowing the physician to ask questions and explain why they may disagree. They may have a good reason as to why the direction they plan to take is best.

4. *Agree* upon next steps. This conversation should be focused on problem-solving, not on arguing or demonstrating your knowledge. Remember the goal is to decide what is best for the patient.

Below is an example of what this may sound like:

Dr. Smith, at our last appointment you mentioned that Jim (the patient) may be starting medication X after today. Based on what you told us, I understand you have had some success treating this disease with medication X. Can you explain to us why you feel it is the best option for Jim as well? I want to be sure we understand it the way you do because I know you want what is best for Jim. (Listen carefully and take diligent notes. If something isn't clear, don't hesitate to clarify.)

Can you tell us more about your past experiences with medication X? How long do you foresee him being on it? What side effects have patients experienced? How quickly do you expect to see results? What negatives are there to taking this drug? What are the long-term effects?

Thank you for explaining your thought process more in-depth to us, Dr. Smith. Jim and I also saw Dr. Kim a few weeks ago for a second opinion. Like you, he is a respected physician within this specialty and has treated many patients with this same disease. First, I wanted to share with you what he told us. (You will then explain and share notes from Dr. Kim's meeting).

Also, I was on (reliable medical website) researching studies about Jim's disease and I found this clinical trial about a new medication that is available (print and bring study). In this clinical trial, patients with Jim's disease took medication Y and had positive results with little side effects. I know we share the same goal, which is to get Jim healthy again. I am bringing this to you, so we can consider all the options. Are you familiar with this clinical trial?

Once you have a moment to review it, I'd like to know what you think about it and if it might be a better option for Jim.

In the conversation above, the advocate shared both the second opinion's plan and results from a clinical trial. Keep in mind this is just an example and you may not have such an arsenal. This example showcases how you might present the information.

The goal of the conversation is to be confident, inquisitive, and respectful. Remember, this discussion should be open and honest, versus accusatory and defensive. For the patient to feel comfortable with the health plan, ask questions until they can see the full picture.

Don't agree to a particular course of action until everyone is aligned. It's important to understand that the patient should play a key role in the decision-making when it comes to their own health.

SWITCHING PROVIDERS

As I stated earlier, I have found that most physicians are caring people who have good hearts. Of course, there will always be some exceptions. In those cases, do not tolerate a physician's bad behavior because of your respect for the profession. If the patient isn't getting the level of care they deserve, it may be time to find a new physician.

Below is an example of when we switched providers to get Meghan the care and attention she needed. Switching providers was not an easy choice. It meant walking away from a physician who was renowned in his field.

> My sister was seeing one of the best lung doctors in the country. No exaggeration. Yet his focus was research. When Meghan first started to see him, we were aware that he didn't see patients as often as other pulmonologists. But because her lung disease was so rare, it was important to all of us that she see a pulmonologist at the top of his field.
>
> From October to February, Meghan's lung treatment was put on hold so that she could focus on battling her cancer. This was because the lung disease required treatment that wasn't permissible while on chemotherapy. Due to the severe decline in her health, we were looking forward to her first post-cancer pulmonology appointment. We were eager to learn the pulmonologist's new plan of attack.
>
> In March, we were told that Meghan beat the cancer. We were elated and ready to get her back to a normal way of living. Recovery now seemed to be in the not-so-distant future. With the right plan in place, we were confident she would regain her health.

Looking back, we were very naïve. When she met with her pulmonologist in March, Meghan discovered there wasn't some grand plan. In fact, after the evaluation, the pulmonologist adjusted her meds slightly and told her he would see her again in June.

Four months between appointments did not sit right with us. But because the pulmonologist was the expert, we went with it. After that meeting, my family was left disheartened and confused.

Remember, Meghan couldn't walk to the bathroom without getting winded. She also was now dependent on an oxygen machine. It was obvious that her health was declining, yet we never questioned her doctor because we believed he knew better. We assumed the medications would do the trick.

In the months after that appointment, over and over we witnessed Meghan's health worsen. She would have difficulty breathing, end up in the ICU, stay in the hospital for weeks, and then fight her way out. She was like a boomerang, spinning back and forth between home and the hospital.

It was a heart-wrenching time for her and our family.

Regardless of her constant hospitalizations, her pulmonologist never made rounds. Certainly, other pulmonologists within the practice visited Meghan when she was hospitalized. Truth be told, it was an uneasy feeling knowing the one in charge of her case wasn't physically seeing what she was going through. We felt she needed a physician who would personally provide her with comfort, support, and direction.

We finally realized it was time for a change. Meghan chose another pulmonologist within the same practice as her primary lung doctor. She had built a nice rapport with one of them who observed her many times in the hospital. He also was easy to get appointments with or call in case of an emergency.

Let me be clear. A new doctor didn't change Meghan's prognosis or the constant hospital visits. Those were inevitable. BO is a nasty and aggressive lung disease. Rather, it meant she received much better care and support. As advocates, we knew this was critical.

Access to the physician was also important for our Badass Advocates team. When Meghan had a health crisis, our family wasn't always sure what action to take. We needed a medical professional to give us clear direction. The higher level of support gave us peace of mind that we were doing right by Meghan. As a Badass Advocate, you won't always have the answers, but you need to be willing to keep asking until you get clear ones.

I do not share this story to bash the renowned pulmonologist. Looking back, there wasn't much he could have done for Meghan's lung disease, and I assume he knew that. He was managing her disease with the proper medications, and that was about all he could do.

I share this story to remind you to constantly be vocal about getting your loved one the care they deserve. To be a Badass Advocate, you must reassess if the approach the physician is taking is the best one. If you have doubts, ask questions, so you aren't left guessing. It's important for advocates and the patient to have a clear understanding of the medical team's thought process. If something doesn't sit right, don't be afraid to challenge the doctor.

Remember you are not committed to one physician. If you live in a small town, your options may be limited. In this case, you may need to trek to the nearest city to find an alternative. If you live in a more suburban or urban area, you should have plenty of physicians to choose from. Either way, if the patient isn't happy with the level of service they are getting, ask others for a referral. When someone is seriously ill, it is imperative that they get the level of care they need.

Inside the hospital, switching providers can be more challenging since you don't proactively "choose" them. The doctor is assigned to the patient's floor or section. But if there is a provider at the hospital who is rude or difficult to work with, you can ask for a replacement.

Before taking next steps, consult the other members of your badass team. It may be helpful to hear their perspective. If the team decides a change would be best, then this kind of request should only be made by one team member. If they are up for the task, the Care Coordinator would be the natural choice. If not, chose a person who can handle the situation with decorum.

It's also important to remind you to not abuse this power. Instead, use it only when it is absolutely necessary. If it is necessary, speak to a supervisor. Then, take the proper steps to get a physician who is more helpful, pleasant, and competent.

On the flip side, this chapter isn't about giving pushback just to give it. There needs to be a certain level of trust in the doctor's decision-making. Questioning every little decision is exhausting and time consuming. If your team is constantly questioning a particular doctor, reassess why there is a lack of trust.

BE RESPECTFUL

We have focused on the importance of being persistent and vocal. Let's now balance that by saying that you must also be respectful. During this time, you or the patient may be grouchy. Feelings of anger, frustration, and fear may be running rampant. No one can blame you for being emotional. However, you will need to learn how to calm your emotions.

I encourage you to look inward and search to understand the root cause of the emotion. The root cause may seem obvious. You are in a dire situation. But dig a little deeper. Try to identify what need isn't being met or what emotion isn't being addressed. Doing some soul searching may help you release the emotional blockage.

Snapping at or being rude to the staff and physicians will not benefit you in any way. See yourself as their teammate, not their opponent. Your job is to support them in helping your loved one. You are *all* part of the same team. Being respectful to the staff and doctors is sage advice for the patient, too.

> Both my father and my sister were patient, kind, and loving souls and, as patients, they had the same demeanor. That's not to say they didn't have their bad days, but they were still kind to their caretakers. Because of how they treated the staff, they were beloved by them.
>
> As a family, we built strong bonds with both nurses and doctors. Consequently, some healthcare providers gave our family special treatment. I remember a week after my sister was released from the ICU, one of the nurses came to visit her during her lunch break. She just wanted to see how Meghan was doing. If you aren't familiar with hospitals, I promise you this isn't the norm.

The point is that medical staff will gravitate towards the patients who are pleasant. They'll try to tolerate the ones who are not. Which bucket do you want to fall in to? Moral of the story: you can be an advocate and be respectful at the same time.

CONCLUSION

If you have been closely involved in your loved one's health journey, then have confidence in what you know. Listen to your gut. If something seems off, don't assume that the physician knows best because they went to medical school. On the other hand, do assume that they are trying their best.

If your goal is to be a Badass Advocate, you must be willing to reach out and speak up. If you feel you aren't getting the answers you need, solicit advice from others and proactively pursue them. Being a Badass Advocate requires being both persistent and respectful. Focus on both, and doors will open.

Remember, this book isn't about how to heal someone who has been diagnosed with a serious disease. This book is about supporting and caring for them while they are in the fight of their lives. If we didn't get Meghan the feeding tube when we did, we may not have had the extra four months of memories that we did. Every extra day with her was a blessing.

BADASS ADVOCATE ACTIONS:

☐ Let your intuition lead you. If something seems wrong, conduct research, ask questions, and voice your concerns.

☐ Proactively seek a second or even third opinion. Obtaining balanced feedback will help you to make sound decisions.

☐ If you reach out to others for advice but don't hear back, don't give up. Pursuing other experts is about getting the answers you need, not the answers you *want*.

☐ Use my four-step technique to effectively and respectfully handle conflict.

☐ Most healthcare professionals are caring and hard-working individuals. If you come across a bad egg, don't tolerate their poor behavior. Find a replacement who is attentive, knowledgeable, and empathetic.

☐ On the flip side, being an advocate does not give you permission to be rude, condescending, or bossy. Stay in control of your emotions, especially anger and frustration.

☐ Maintain a mindset that the support team and the medical professionals are one team. Focus on working *together* to help your loved one heal.

"The good physician treats the disease; the great physician treats the patient who has the disease."

~ *Dr. William Osler*

A founder of Johns Hopkins Hospital who created the first residency program.

Ask Strong Questions

One skill that will help you in your quest to be a Badass Advocate is to ask good questions.

When it comes to asking questions, some of us are more inquisitive and easily think of questions. Yet others may need more time to contemplate and come back with questions. If knowing what to ask is more challenging for you, developing your questioning skills will be an important step to becoming a Badass Advocate.

In this chapter, I will explain how I used my professional experience as a pharmaceutical sales representative to ask better questions on behalf of my sister. I will teach you how to be deliberate in the types of questions you ask, as well as some simple techniques that will help you get the answers you need.

You will also learn about how to compile a strong list of questions and when to ask the tough ones. Ultimately, asking solid questions is a skill that will strengthen your advocacy. You will begin to see how your conversations can evolve and be more informative. Gaining more knowledge of your loved one's case will help you feel empowered.

Hospital Rounds

It is always best to have a support team member present at the hospital, but unfortunately, this is not always possible. Our support team also faced this issue, and it posed several challenges for us.

When Meghan was in the hospital, we seemed to have unfortunate timing. Many times, Meghan would be by herself when the physician visited. This was an issue because between the meds and her health condition, she had a tendency to be confused. Being in an altered state meant we couldn't rely on her to ask critical questions or remember detailed information given by the physicians.

We also realized that doctor rounds were an opportune time to speak with the hospitalists. If you aren't familiar with the term "rounds," it is when hospital staff (doctors, nurses, etc.) visit patient rooms to discuss the patient's case. If your loved one is at a teaching hospital, residents will also be present.

The first time Meghan was hospitalized, no one told us that we should be present for rounds. Then, after a few sleepovers in the hospital, we realized that rounds gave us a prime opportunity to easily meet with her doctors. Rounds always took place at the same time each day—first thing in the morning, right after the shift change at 7:00 AM. If you came after 8:00 AM, you most likely missed your chance.

This was a key piece of information. During the day, when we had questions, it was more challenging to find a physician. Of course, the nurses would call the doctor if we asked. But many times, it took a while for them to get to the room, and if it wasn't urgent, it often wasn't worth the hassle.

If you need to speak with a physician, don't hesitate to request one. We did many times. But sometimes our questions weren't pressing, so we would wait until the next morning.

During rounds, ask if you can listen as the doctors review your loved one's case. What they share can be eye-opening. If your loved one's disease is complicated, it may be a real opportunity to learn and understand it better.

If the physician is comfortable with you listening, my recommendation is to wake up early and get ready before rounds begin. Once rounds begin, you can stand quietly in the background, listen attentively, and make note of the questions you want to ask.

After the staff finishes their discussion, then you can speak to the attending physician—the doctor who is responsible for the visiting patient and overseeing their treatment. There will be multiple attendings tending to your loved one's care. I recommend getting to know each of them, so you can build a relationship and feel comfortable asking them questions.

Carefully consider which questions you ask in front of the patient as some answers can be upsetting, so you may want to ask certain questions in a private setting instead. Otherwise, you can wait until the doctor comes into the patient's room, and all discuss the case together.

Remember that the patient needs to give medical staff permission to discuss their health information with you. They may be more private and not want other people to have access to this information. I recommend having an open discussion with your loved one. All the while maintain the mindset that disclosure is at their discretion, and they are the primary decision-maker.

ORGANIZE A LIST

Now that we've explored the best time to ask questions, let's focus on how to be well-prepared for that meeting. Before you meet with any doctor (whether in the hospital or otherwise), you should compile a list of questions.

First, you will need to ask for input from both the patient and the support team. My family typically came up with a list via text messaging, which was an easy way for us to organize.

Let's say a support team member is visiting the patient in the hospital. They discover that they will have the opportunity to speak to one of the physicians. That team member should immediately notify the group of this opportunity. Then the group should begin to compile a list of questions.

If the next time you will speak to the physician is during rounds, then collect questions ahead of time. Preparation is key.

When your loved one is at home, prepare for doctor's appointments the same way. If they see multiple specialists, then inform your army which one the patient will be seeing. The specialty could affect the types of questions people want to ask.

BRAINSTORMING IS POWERFUL

Allowing the team to see others' questions naturally generates a brainstorming session. One question can spark a new thought and so on. Getting input from the group is a powerful practice. Brainstorming as a team will allow you to generate a more concentrated list of questions.

Remember to include the patient as well, even though they may be overwhelmed or distracted. When a physician is present, the patient may forget what they want to say. Preparing them ahead of time takes the pressure off them. It also gives them time to think about what questions they want answered.

If your loved one is clear-minded and up for the task, they should be leading the conversation. You can then pepper in the team's questions when appropriate. Remember it is their health journey, so they should be in charge. Feeling in charge of something is good for someone who may be feeling like they are not in control of much.

On the other hand, if the patient isn't coherent or up for the task, the team member who is present will need to take charge. As I mentioned before, be mindful of talking about the patient as if they aren't present. Talking over them can make them feel insignificant, which is the last thing you want.

ACCESSIBILITY

You also should maintain a comprehensive list of questions and ensure that everyone on the team can access that list. You can use an app, like Flock, where you can create a group chat room to share questions, updates, photos, and more.

Another option is to do what my family did—create a group text message chain. We named ours Team Meg.

When it was my turn to ask questions of the physician, I had a system for collecting the questions. Before meeting the physician, I would reference the group text and copy and paste the questions into the Notes app on my phone. I transferred the questions beforehand, so I was prepared. My fear was if I referenced the questions within the text message chain, some would get lost in the mix.

Saving them in one place also guaranteed every suggested question would be asked. I reviewed them as they came in and eliminated duplicates. When the doctor was present, I could calmly and easily find them.

Figure out a system that works best for you. The most important piece is to be sure that you have the questions with you during the meeting. The last thing you want is for the questions to be written on a piece of scratch paper that was left at home on the counter.

TYPES OF QUESTIONS

Let's dive into the different types of questions you can ask, how to use them to your advantage, and how to get the answers you really want.

OPEN-ENDED QUESTIONS

Every year I teach new sales reps how to ask questions. I explain that questions fall into two categories: open or closed.

Open-ended questions start with "who," "what," "when," "where," "why," and "how." Open-ended questions are helpful for gaining more information. Beginning your questions with these words will naturally encourage a more in-depth response.

Closed-ended questions, on the other hand, begin with "are," "do," "have," "is," and "will." These types of questions elicit a "yes" or "no" response, meaning answers are less in-depth.

Someone who tends to be talkative may expand on their answer, regardless. However, if you want to gain more information, focus on using open-ended questions.

Asking open-ended questions can be challenging because they can feel invasive. In addition, closed-ended questions allow the questioner to control the conversation, whereas open-ended questions can make us feel like we are putting someone on the spot.

If you have never paid attention to the type of questions you ask, I encourage you to begin doing so. You can easily practice this skill with friends, family, and strangers.

To create a solid list of open-ended questions for your loved one's physicians, start by jotting down as many questions as you can. At first, try not to edit your thinking. Scribble away.

Now that your list is complete, turn any closed-ended questions into open-ended ones. You usually can identify closed-ended questions using the first word.

Once you've identified the closed-ended questions, you can reword them so that they start with "who," "what," "when," "where," "why," and "how." Most likely you will need to play around with the wording, so it makes sense. Below is an example:

> *Closed-Ended:* "Do you recommend that she walks daily?"

> *Open-Ended:* "What kind of exercise should she be doing? How often and how long should she exercise?"

In the example above, the person asking the closed-ended question assumes that the healthcare provider wants the patient to walk. If the healthcare provider sticks to only answering the question, they might respond "no." The discussion could then end. But asking an open-ended question could encourage the healthcare provider to give more information. They can respond how they see fit. They are not locked into only focusing on walking.

Open-ended questions will allow you to get a better understanding of the patient's situation. Closed-ended questions tend to force the listener in a certain direction. Open-ended questions may also make sure that the provider doesn't unintentionally leave out key information.

In the above example, the open-ended question opens the door for many answers. The provider can give you a list of exercise options. The follow-up question allows the provider to give even further detailed information. He may expand on how often and how long they want the patient to exercise.

Asking good questions like these is a great way to advocate for your loved one. It will help you to receive more detailed and clearer answers.

CLARIFYING AND CONFIRMING

Throughout these conversations, you'll also want to pepper in clarifying and confirming questions. Unfortunately, preparing for these ahead of time is not as easy. These types of questions are based on what the person is saying in the moment. If listening to others isn't a strength, then asking clarifying and confirming questions may be challenging. Paying close attention to what the speaker is saying is key.

Let me explain how clarifying and confirming questions can be used to your advantage.

CLARIFYING QUESTIONS

Clarifying questions allow you to further understand what the other person means when they speak subjectively.

An example of this would be if the physician says, "Your loved one should be eating a healthier diet." The subjective term is "healthier." We all have different interpretations of what "healthier" means. That could mean eating less red meat, eating a vegan diet, cutting out sugar completely, or avoiding alcohol. Because there are so many ways to interpret the word "healthier," you need to clarify.

A good follow-up question to this statement would be, "Doctor, how do you define 'healthier'?" or "What set of guidelines can you provide for us, so we can support our loved one in following a 'healthier' diet?" Most of us would hear what the physician recommended and assume we knew what he meant by "healthy." In reality, our thoughts or opinions may not be aligned with the doctor's.

The trick is to listen for a subjective word (e.g. healthier) and then form a question around it. This will help you to better understand what the person means. Notice, I kept both questions open-ended. This helped me to gain a better understanding of what the doctor meant by "healthier." Again, open-ended questions will help you to gain more information and clarity.

CONFIRMING QUESTIONS

Confirming questions are another useful tool to help you gain accurate information and check your comprehension. You will use confirming questions when you are unclear about what the physician is telling you.

To determine when to ask confirming questions, tune into your gut. If you feel a tinge of confusion when the physician is speaking, then begin asking confirming questions. You'll want to continue asking confirming questions until you are clear. Don't let embarrassment stop you from asking questions. Remind yourself that this is what a Badass Advocate would do.

A confirming question could be, "Doctor, are you saying that my mother should only be taking that medication once a day versus twice a day like she was before? Am I understanding you correctly?" Confirming questions can be either closed or open-ended.

Below are some examples of how to start a confirming question:

"To confirm, are you telling me..."

"If I understand you correctly, do you feel that..."

"Let me see if I understand what you are saying..."

When it comes to advocating for your loved one, the last thing you want to do is make assumptions. Your assumption could be completely wrong, which could be disastrous.

ACTIVE LISTENING

Asking questions is one skill but listening to someone's response is another. First, try not to formulate a response while the doctor is talking. If you don't focus on listening to what the other person is telling you, it's a waste of everyone's time. Stephen Covey, author and influential speaker, has a great quote about listening:

"Most people do not listen with the intent to understand; they listen with the intent to reply."

Many times, when we ask a question, we are so busy thinking about what *we* want to say next that we don't listen to the answer. Writing down the question ahead of time will help you to develop the skill of listening. You'll notice that you will be less concerned about remembering what you need to ask next. Your list will serve as your memory.

Focusing on clarifying and confirming will also help you to develop stronger listening skills. This happens because you will be forced to listen to what the physician is telling you. The key is to focus on every word the person says. If they are giving you a lot of information and you can't keep up, ask them if they can pause for a moment while you make notes.

If you can actively listen, you can ask better questions. In turn, the conversation will be more informative. Like anything else, it takes practice to develop good listening and questioning skills. The good news is you can practice this skill with anyone you meet.

ASK THE TOUGH QUESTIONS

My last piece of advice is for those of you who are dealing with a critically ill patient. If their health seems to be declining and no one has given a recent prognosis, you will need to take the reins and muster up the courage to ask the tough questions. Initiating this conversation is burdensome, but necessary. In my experience, having a clear picture of what's on the horizon will save you from future regrets.

> I was only 20 years old when my father died. Since then, one of my biggest regrets was not asking the physician about my dad's prognosis. I was completely blindsided by his death. I knew he was sick but believed he would eventually get better.

After he died, I had to deal with feelings of regret and guilt—regret for unfinished conversations and guilt for not spending more time with him.

This shame influenced me to change my behavior when Meghan got sick. I was determined to be deliberate in how I spent my time. I needed to get answers to some serious questions.

Was it necessary for me to constantly jump on a plane, or was everything not as urgent as we suspected? Were we being dramatic when we worried she was going to die, or were the doctors hinting at what was to come? Did I need to mentally prepare myself for losing her, or could I hold out hope that we would grow old together? Did I need to talk to her about end-of-life decisions, or could I continue to convince her she would get through this?

So many unanswered questions led to a lot of anxiety and fear.

I was scared and nervous to ask about her prognosis. But I had to know what was ahead, so I could make educated decisions and mentally prepare myself and my family. I decided to separately ask three physicians about her prognosis. I reached out to two attendings and Dr. Aron. I knew the prognosis was true when all three doctors gave similar answers.

Each response was disheartening. In essence, they said, "It's challenging to predict an exact amount of time a patient has left to live. For Meghan, six months is most likely, but unfortunately, if she catches an infection, it could kill her."

My heart sunk. What my mind had been warning my heart was true. All I could focus on was "six months." That meant she most likely wouldn't live until the end of the year.

One attending also added, "Hey, but you never know, maybe she will beat the odds and beat this thing." His optimism was kind.

My heart wanted to believe this to be fact, but my brain knew it was probably not likely. Although I anticipated their answer, it was still shocking to hear.

Hearing it was necessary. It allowed us to make informed decisions.

I hope you don't find yourself in the same situation, but if you do, I encourage you to get the answers you need. This is not easy, but you can do it. I promise, you won't regret it in the end.

RECEIVING THE WORST NEWS

If you receive dreaded news, then you will need to shift your mindset. Up until this point, you have been in fight mode. You've been doing all that you can to get your loved one the care they deserve so that they can battle their disease and get well.

If the prognosis is bad, you need to tell yourself that it is not a reflection of your valiant efforts. Remind yourself of that—regularly. You can do everything "right" and still end up in this place.

In addition, remember that you can—and should—still be a Badass Advocate, but your duties will now be a bit different. Your focus will shift from disease-targeted care to comfort-focused care. You will now concentrate on helping the patient live their remaining days pain free and in peace. This time will be one of the most challenging parts of your journey.

Although your focus has changed, your role as an advocate is no less important. In fact, your responsibilities may be heightened because the patient will not be the only one who needs help. What will begin to unfold will be difficult for everyone involved, including you.

Once the physician has informed the patient of their prognosis, it will be critical for you to support the patient by helping them get the emotional support they need. The patient will need reassurance that they can openly voice their fears and receive empathy in return.

Whether they confide in you or someone else, like a palliative care doctor, is not important. What is important is that they have the opportunity to open up to someone who can be sensitive to what they are dealing with. The last thing you want is for the patient's anxiety and fears to be dismissed or minimized.

You should also speak to your loved one about who they want around during their final days. They may not want certain people to see them in this condition. This is a part of their inner peace.

Let's also not forget about the impact this news has on family members, friends, and you.

First, I vehemently advocate for being forthright with everyone who is closely involved with the patient, even young children. Keeping the patient's prognosis from others is a bad idea with negative consequences.

I know from first-hand experience that telling people that their loved one will not live much longer is not easy. In fact, it's heart-wrenching and takes a lot of courage. I don't wish this task upon anyone. However, if you find yourself in this position, realize that your actions can be life-changing for someone else.

If you or others decide to withhold the truth, understand that you are making a major life decision for someone else. You are choosing to take away their opportunity to do what *they* need to in order to make peace with their loved one's death. Speaking from personal experience, this can cause years of pain and anger (and the need for lots of therapy).

It is fair to say that all of you will need help accepting your new reality. It may be difficult to wrap your brain around the unimaginable. Even though the patient is alive, the grieving process has, in a way, already begun. Everyone will deal with that in their own way.

Last, it is important for me to share that this time also poses an opportunity for survivors to fulfill their own needs. The last thing anyone should live with is lifelong regrets. Encourage others, especially children, to say what they feel is necessary because they may not get this opportunity again.

This situation is a harsh reality that you may not want to face, and that is why I am addressing it now. I hope that by bringing it to your attention, you can begin to face your fears and address what lies ahead.

SPEAKING TO CHILDREN

Trying to protect a child from the pain of a parent being diagnosed with a serious illness is common and understandable. However, according to MD Anderson Cancer Center, research shows that:

- A parent's cancer diagnosis affects a child whether or not the child is informed of the condition.

- Anxiety levels are higher in children who aren't informed about their parent's condition, compared to children where the issue is discussed.

- For parents of teenagers, an important aspect of coping is ongoing communication between the teens and their parents during the course of the illness.

The point is that "honest, age-appropriate communication is best." To further support parents and their children, MD Anderson has created a program called KIWI (Kids Inquire, We Inform). KIWI focuses on helping children and teens to cope with a parent's cancer by providing tools and training for parents and caregivers. Visit their website[2] for more information on the KIWI program.

Speaking to a child about a loved one's chronic illness or impending death can be incredibly difficult. But you don't have to go it alone. There are many resources to support you and the child during this sad and confusing time.

One important step is to reach out to the child's school to inform them of what is happening. Making the teachers and school counselors aware will give the child support during the day. It will also give them added comfort to know that they can speak to someone if they get upset while at school.

Furthermore, those in charge can be on the lookout for changes in behavior. The school can further support the family by alerting them if any issues or concerns arise.

Dr. Jennifer Aron, who deals with this situation often, also suggests contacting the child life team at your loved one's hospital. Child life

---

[2] https://www.mdanderson.org/patients-family/diagnosis-treatment/patient-support/kids-inquire-we-inform.html

specialists[3] are clinically trained professionals who work with children dealing with traumatic life events. They provide children with emotional support and helpful tools when facing serious illness, disability, and loss.

Many organizations also support children *after* their loved one dies. Sometimes it helps to know you are not the only kid dealing with the death of a parent, sibling, or close relative.

For more resources on how to support children dealing with loss or a loved one's serious illness, go to www.badassadvocate.com/resources.

CONCLUSION

Asking strong questions is a powerful tool advocates can use. If the techniques I've discussed are new to you, practice using them with family and friends. Asking good questions is a skill that can be easily learned.

If your loved one's situation seems to be taking a turn for the worse, it may be time to have a heart-to-heart with them and their physician. Assuming the patient has given medical staff permission to share medical information with you, it is best if you understand what the future holds. If the patient is not going to live much longer, take the appropriate steps to get them, their loved ones, and yourself the emotional support all of you need.

---

[3] https://www.childlife.org/the-child-life-profession

Badass Advocate Actions:

- ☐ Be present during rounds because they are the best time to speak to hospitalists.

- ☐ Proactively brainstorm with the support team and patient to come up with a list of questions *prior* to rounds or doctor's appointments. Having a strong list will help you get the information you need.

- ☐ Actively listen during key conversations so you may leave feeling fully informed.

- ☐ Convert closed-ended questions to open-ended ones. This will allow you to gain more informative answers.

- ☐ Use clarifying questions to further understand what you are being told and confirming questions to ensure your take-aways are accurate.

- ☐ Muster up the courage to ask the uncomfortable end-of-life questions. These questions will help you to make informed decisions while your loved one is still alive.

- ☐ If children are closely related to the patient, have honest conversations and get them the extra support they will need.

♡

"The biggest lie I tell myself is, 'I don't need to write that down. I'll remember it.'"

~*Unknown*

Badass Strategy #4
Prevent Forgetfulness

The last chapter examined effective questioning techniques you can use to get more in-depth answers from medical staff. Once you develop this skill, you will then need to remember everything the staff tells you. If that last sentence gives you anxiety, don't worry. I have a solution.

In a stressful situation, remembering a barrage of new information may be a challenge. Furthermore, the medical advice you receive is vital, so you don't want to miss or forget a word. This is why my family recorded conversations with healthcare providers—a practice I believe is critical for being a Badass Advocate.

If you take only one piece of advice from this book, this should be it. Recording conversations with each provider was one of the best things we did. The reason why it isn't listed as Badass Strategy #1 is because to be the best Badass Advocate, you should implement strategies 1 through 3 first. It makes the most sense.

GAIN PERMISSION

Before you press record, understand that you *must* get permission from the patient. A patient's healthcare information is private, so it is up to the patient if they wish for it to be recorded and shared.

When you ask for permission, explain to the patient why you are making these recordings. Hopefully, once they see the positives, they will give you permission. If not, do your best to take diligent notes and keep track of pertinent information.

Once the patient agrees, you will then need to ask the medical professional for permission. Remember to ask for permission at *the start of each meeting.* Explain that the recordings serve two main purposes. One, they can help the patient remember the conversation, and, two, they can keep team members informed. Still, some physicians may be hesitant for you to record them due to fears of a potential lawsuit. If this is the case, plan on taking meticulous notes.

Speaking of lawsuits, recording the physician is *not* intended for entrapment, manipulation, or blame. Remember the medical staff is part of your team. That means the recordings should help you to work better together by allowing you to clarify information and follow up with questions.

One of the most important aspects of being an advocate is protecting your sick loved one. This doesn't mean searching for wrong-doings. It means paying close attention, so you can prevent mistakes from happening.

Mistakes can range from minimal to life-threatening. One reason advocates are so important is that they can help catch and prevent mistakes. If you don't think mistakes can happen to your loved one, think again.

Over an eight-year period, Johns Hopkin's collected medical-related death data. They found that in the U.S. over 250,000 deaths per year are due to medical errors. This makes medical errors the third leading cause of deaths.[4]

---

[4] https://hub.jhu.edu/2016/05/03/medical-errors-third-leading-cause-of-death/

I don't share this information to scare you or imply that doctors are incompetent. I share these findings to prove the seriousness and importance of patient advocacy. Be knowledgeable, pay attention, and speak up when necessary.

Out of everything we did, I felt like recording the conversations was the single most important step we took to strengthen our team. Those recordings helped each one of us to be accurately informed. This meant that as Meghan's soldiers, we each understood what was happening and what needed to be done. Eliminating the risk of misinterpretation allowed us to stay aligned. Here is how we did it.

RECORDING CONVERSATIONS

Recording providers may be a simple and effective way to strengthen your team, but the key to success is being consistent. Recording conversations should be an expectation for any person who witnesses doctor conversations.

If you have a smart phone, most likely it has an app that will record sound. For example, the iPhone has an app called "Voice Memos." When you open the app, click on the red button at the bottom to record. When you want the recording to stop, simply click on the red button again. Apps on the Android phone system work similarly. Practice a bit with the app before you use it to record your first conversation with a doctor.

To make sure the recording is clear, hold the microphone towards those who are speaking. It doesn't need to be in their face, but it should be within a few feet of them. I also recommend setting it on a flat surface to decrease background noise. Holding the phone in your hand can generate a lot of extra noise that makes the recording harder to understand.

Once the recording is finished, change the title of the file to include who the conversation was with. If more detail is needed, include the subject of the conversation and date (e.g., Dr. Smith, Picc Line Update, 03.01.20). Titles make it easy to reference the recordings when needed.

Always make sure the date is in the title of your file, as it is a key piece of information you'll need in the future. Please note, the iPhone's Voice Memo app will automatically note the date.

After you've titled your recording, you'll then want to share it with the patient and members of the support team. Again, make sure you only send it to people the patient has approved to receive such information.

Keep in mind that longer recordings may be too large to send via text or email. In that case, you can upload them to a cloud-based, file-sharing site. Many offer free versions, including Dropbox, Google Drive, and WeTransfer.

Now that you understand how to set up the recordings, let's talk about the purpose they serve.

PATIENT-DOCTOR MEETINGS

There may be times when no support team members are present at physician meetings. If the patient is coherent and has a cell phone, they can easily record their own conversations. If possible, I recommend calling them before the meeting to remind them.

Having the patient record their own conversations is helpful for several reasons. First, it allows the support team members to know exactly what was said in their absence. I don't recommend depending on the patient to reiterate the conversation. Most likely they won't remember every detail and asking them to recount it may be draining or even upsetting.

During the meetings when team members aren't present, the patient can still ask questions from your team's pre-arranged list. A second benefit is that recordings will help you verify that the patient did indeed ask the planned questions. If they did, you will then be able to hear the doctor's answers. If they didn't ask all of your questions, then you will know that you need to follow up with that physician.

Last, the patient may have brain fog due to their medical condition or medication. Another benefit is that while you are listening, you may notice little interaction on the patient's behalf. This exact situation happened with Meghan, and it gave us a clue that something was off. It wasn't a benefit of the recordings that we expected, but it worked.

COMMUNICATION

Recording conversations also helps to keep the support team aligned.

I can't tell you how many times I have walked away from a sales call where both the sales rep and I heard completely different things. Listeners will interpret conversations in their own way. In turn, they may relay conflicting information to others.

Remember playing "telephone" or "whisper down the lane" as a kid? How likely was it for the last person to repeat the exact same phrase as the first person? Not likely. What often happened was the last person would receive a jumbled message. Words would be missing or replaced with other, similar-sounding words.

"Whisper down the lane" was a fun game that taught a great life lesson. When humans pass along a message, they unintentionally put their own spin on it. And as it continues to be passed on, the message becomes more twisted.

This is why recording conversations is so helpful. It greatly reduces the likelihood of poor communication.

REPLAY

Recordings also enable each team member to listen to the conversation at whatever time best suits them. If necessary, they can replay the parts of the conversation that they find most relevant. You may discover that you each tend to focus on different topics or moments. This is natural and also helpful—it enables you to widen the perspective and leverage the different insights of the team.

In addition, the Care Coordinator can use these recordings to assist with note-taking. They can jot down key points in their notebook as they listen. They can pause as needed and capture the information they need most for future reference.

VERIFICATION

Caretakers have a lot on their minds. So, when a healthcare provider is giving important information, you may feel overwhelmed. A big benefit of the recordings is the playback feature. When needed, you can go back into the archives and verify what the healthcare provider said.

Or, during the meeting you may feel you understand what the doctor is telling you. But later upon reflection, you may feel unclear. Recordings will allow you to double check.

Our mom was Meghan's main Care Coordinator. In that role, she would often re-listen to the recordings. It helped her to keep information straight and confirm what she thought she heard.

CONNECTION

Recordings are a great way for those who live far away to feel connected to the patient and what is going on with their care. Before sharing any recordings, confirm with the patient who they approve of hearing them. We shared the recordings only with our immediate family members.

Usually, when I called for updates, I received the highlights reel. That meant I would also miss out on issues that people felt were less significant or more nuanced. This was understandable. Taking care of a sick loved one is physically and emotionally draining. Rehashing the conversation was the last thing they wanted to do.

On the other hand, I wanted to understand what was going on and was hoping to hear specific details. Instead, I was getting pieces of information here and there. It was confusing. To no one's fault, I felt disconnected and of no good use.

That is when it occurred to me that we needed to start recording conversations. Having the recordings took the pressure off my family to re-explain details. At the same time, they allowed me to feel well informed.

KEEPING TRACK

If your loved one has a long battle ahead, the recordings may serve as a way to keep track of their progress. Obviously, there is a medical chart with the details of their case. But not every conversation and minute detail will be included.

If you have your loved one's permission, you can share the recordings with other physicians. This will make those doctors aware of what the primary team is advising. The clearer the communication, the better.

Video Recording

In certain cases, it may be better to use the video function. An example of this is when a medical professional is demonstrating something to you. We only used video once, but looking back, there may have been other times when video could have been helpful.

> I mentioned earlier that at one point Meghan had a feeding tube. The first time it was inserted, she was in the hospital. But once she returned home, the support team would be responsible for it and would need to know how to switch out the feedings and keep the tube sterile.

> Ensuring the caretaker could keep the feeding tube sterile was vital to Meghan's health. Contamination could cause a serious infection and kill her.

> The day Meghan was discharged, the feeding tube company sent a representative to the hospital to teach us how to use the machine and change out the feeding tube. I was the only team member there when he arrived. This was unfortunate since I didn't live locally, and I knew I wouldn't be responsible for her feedings every day. It would most likely be our mom or Meghan's husband.

> Meghan and I agreed that recording a video of the demonstration would be helpful. Like the audio recordings, the video made it easy to watch, replay, and learn.

Conclusion

Recording conversations with medical professionals can be an incredibly useful tool. After all, supporting a seriously ill patient can be overwhelming and a lot to manage. The recordings will help you to manage the situation better and keep the team aligned.

The main goal of being an advocate is to ensure the patient receives the best care available. But, this may not be as easy as it seems. Information gets lost, mistakes can happen, and new medical issues may arise. An advocate plays a critical role because they witness all the moving parts. Putting smart practices into place, like this one, will give you the superpowers you need to be a Badass Advocate.

Badass Advocate Actions:

☐ Record conversations with medical professionals so your badass team can stay up-to-date on the patient's case.

☐ Prior to recording, gain permission from both the patient and the provider.

☐ Use recordings to verify information, stay informed, and keep the team aligned.

☐ Teach patients how to record conversations and get them in the habit of doing so. You can further support by listening to the recordings and following up if necessary.

"The greatest enemy to knowledge is not ignorance. It is the illusion of knowledge."

~ *Stephen Hawking*

A world-renowned theoretical physicist, cosmologist, and author who was paralyzed most of his life due to ALS.

Gain & Apply Powerful Knowledge

Gaining information through effective questioning and recording conversations are key elements to advocating. But if you aren't well-versed in the relevant medical jargon, you will have a limited understanding of what all of these conversations really mean.

Don't worry! You don't have to put yourself through a mini-medical school to be informed. Instead, focus your attention on what relates to your loved one's case so that you can be knowledgeable about *their* situation.

In this chapter, I'll share with you some of the medical terms I learned and used most often. I'll also share with you questions you can ask to learn what is relevant. Keep in mind: each person's situation is different, so you'll need to conduct some of your own research.

First and foremost, take the time to educate yourself on what is relevant to the patient's illness. The best way to do this is to be observant. Listen to the medical staff and pay close attention to what terms they use most often.

If your loved one is in the hospital, a good time to learn is during shift changes because that is when nurses review the patient's case. It's a sort of "passing the baton" ritual. They recap all that happened in the past 12 hours, and these conversations are typically very informative.

During shift changes when Meghan was in the hospital, I would pay close attention to the terminology the nurses used.

Some terms I could understand using common sense, but with others, I had no idea what they were talking about.

I realized that one way I could further support both Meghan and the attending staff was by becoming more knowledgeable. I also knew that to get the most information possible, I should ask open-ended questions because those questions encourage people to speak more openly and share more of their insights.

Here are some of the key terms that I learned that helped empower me the most.

VITAL SIGNS MONITOR

Familiarize yourself with the vital signs monitor. The vital signs monitor is a small machine located next to the patient and directly connected to them through various wires. The machine constantly checks the patient's "vitals," including their heart rate, blood pressure, oxygen saturation, respiration, and temperature. The machine will also set off an alarm if one of these vital signs becomes worrisome.

As an advocate, it is empowering to understand the various numbers and what they mean. Furthermore, you'll want to know your loved one's ideal ranges.

Keep in mind: sometimes the ideal ranges for a healthy patient are not the same as the ideal ranges for a sick person. If you understand your loved one's ideal numbers, then you'll know when something is wrong.

You'll notice that the vital signs monitor alarms often. This can be both annoying and upsetting. But if you understand the numbers and how the monitor works, then you can take appropriate action.

In some cases, the alarm will falsely indicate an emergency while in others you will need to urgently call a nurse. A non-emergency situation could be something like needing to readjust a wire to remove a kink. This seems to happen often since wires can get caught up in a bedridden patient. Once you learn the signs that it is a kink and not an emergency, you can gently move the patient's arm and untangle the wires.

To help you begin to understand the vital signs monitor, you can ask the nurse the following questions:

- What does _____ [specific acronym] mean?

- What is the ideal number for [specific vital sign] when it comes to a healthy patient?

- What is the ideal number for [specific vital sign] when it comes to my loved one?

- When there isn't a nurse in the room and the machine starts beeping, what can I do to help? Is there an easy way to know if it's a kink in the wire versus an emergency?

- How can we help get the [specific vital sign] back to where it needs to be?

Aim to use positive language. The last two questions assume there is something you can do to help. It's a good idea to put the nurse or doctor in the mindset that you are willing to support their efforts and that you want to be part of the care team.

PATIENT EVALUATION SCALES

If your loved one becomes hospitalized, you may hear about the AVPU or ACDU scales and NEWS values. Hospitals may use either the AVPU or ACDU scales to evaluate the patient's mental responsiveness while they may use the NEWS values to assess the patient's vital signs.

These ratings help medical staff determine if the patient needs immediate medical attention. Understanding these scales means you can use them in or out of the hospital to call for help.

AVPU & ACDU

AVPU stands for **A**lert, **V**oice, **P**ain, and **U**nresponsive. Each letter represents a different level of responsiveness.

- *Alert* means the patient is aware of their surroundings and able to respond to commands.

- *Voice* means the patient is verbally responsive.

- *Pain* means the patient only responds to a painful prod by an examiner.

- *Unresponsive* means the patient doesn't respond to commands or prods at all.

A	The patient is awake
V	The patient responds to verbal stimulation
P	The patient responds to painful stimulation
U	The patient is completely unresponsive

Like AVPU, ACDU is a four-point scale that assesses the patient's level of consciousness. **ACDU** stands for **A**lertness, **C**onfusion, **D**rowsiness and **U**nresponsiveness. The levels are self-explanatory and similar to the AVPU scale.

Your loved one's hospital may use either scale. I recommend asking the staff to find out which scale they reference. Knowing this allows you to understand what the medical staff is talking about and your loved one's status.

Keep in mind: you don't have to wait until your loved one gets hospitalized to use them. You also don't need any formal training to use them, and they can help you recognize if it is time to call 911.

News Scales

As mentioned earlier, the National Early Warning Score (NEWS) scale is another evaluation tool used within hospital systems. It assesses six physiological parameters, including temperature, systolic blood pressure, pulse rate, oxygen saturation, respiratory rate, and level of consciousness.

Because you need to know the patient's vital signs for NEWS, it can be a little more complicated. But if the patient is hooked up to a vital sign monitor, you should be able to use this evaluation tool as well. If you wish to understand this scale more in-depth, head to the Royal College of Physicians[5] website for more information. To make it easier for you, I have also posted a link on my website www.badassadvocate.com/resources.

---

[5] https://www.rcplondon.ac.uk/projects/outputs/national-early-warning-score-news-2

We have all heard the saying "knowledge is power." Yet, simply *having* the knowledge isn't what makes you powerful; it's how you *apply* that knowledge that makes the impact. Once you start putting your learnings into action, you'll be more confident and effective.

TAKE ACTION WHEN NEEDED

If you understand the vital signs and what is an emergency, you can act when needed. I took action based on my own knowledge while visiting Meghan one day in the hospital.

Like most days, she was resting in her bed. Her eyes were closed, and she looked peaceful. I was quietly working in the chair beside her bed. Apart from the beeping of machines, the room was silent.

In a nanosecond, the peaceful setting turned into chaos. Suddenly Meghan's heart monitor started to alarm. With a panicked look on her face, she blurted out "Erin, I feel like my heart is racing." I glanced over at her heart monitor and observed the numbers rapidly rising. I fearfully watched as her heart rate rose to almost 180 while she remained sedentary in bed.

I was confused and frightened. What was happening?

To give you context, a healthy resting heart rate is between 60 – 100. But I knew during her illness, her heart rate was typically on the higher end of that range. However, a heart rate of 180 for a sedentary person is alarming.

She looked terrified, and her eyes pleaded for me to help. I did my best to remain calm, so I would not cause her more distress. I leaned over and pushed the call button, which was resting on her bed. We waited for what seemed like an eternity for a response.

I hastily strode to the door while maintaining eye contact with the monitor. I then looked in Meghan's eyes and gently assured her she would be okay and that I would get a nurse.

I was afraid to leave her alone, so I stepped into the hallway to see if I could grab a nurse passing by. The hallway was frustratingly quiet. I was forced to make a choice: either I run for help or sit and hope a nurse answers the call.

In a last attempt to get help and not leave her alone, I pushed the bed's alert button. No response. It was time to make a move.

I assured Meghan I'd be right back. Once I was out of Meghan's sight, I sprinted down the hallway to get help. I finally found a nurse and frantically requested she come with me.

Once we got to the room, she evaluated Meghan and checked the monitors. As the nurse was checking Meghan out, we watched in amazement as her heart rate began to go down. It declined as quickly as it rose.

Now that her heart rate was back to normal, we could finally take a deep breath. I'm explaining how this scene took place in slow motion, but in reality, all this happened in a matter of seconds.

The nurse reassured us she was fine now, and she would call the on-call doctor to check on Meghan. In the meantime, she said I should keep an eye on her and call for help if it happened again.

Later, the attending told us that her racing heart rate was just a freak thing. He explained that sometimes this happens, and there is no clear explanation for it. But he warned that if it continued to happen, there might be another underlying issue.

We were lucky. It never happened again.

I share this story so that you can understand the power of knowledge. I knew Meghan's normal heart rate and how dangerous a heart rate of 180 was to her health. If you understand what equals an emergency and what doesn't, you will know when to call for help.

Conclusion

Educating yourself about your loved one's disease and relevant medical terms can be powerful. As you gain more knowledge, you can ask more effective questions, rely less on others, and fight for the patient when needed. Encourage your army to do the same and support one another during this learning journey. Ultimately, this newfound knowledge will help the team to be better advocates.

Badass Advocate Actions:

- ☐ Know when shift changes take place and aim to be present. When you are present, focus on listening, learning, and asking questions.

- ☐ Educate yourself by understanding the patient's disease and their specific health information.

- ☐ Familiarize yourself with the evaluation scales used by the hospital. Then, team up with the staff and act when needed.

- ☐ If the patient is homebound, use the evaluation scales to assess the patient's health status and determine if they need further medical assistance.

- ☐ Stay well-informed so you can be an influential advocate. Knowing about your loved one's condition can reduce stress and allow you to advocate for them in critical situations.

- ☐ You may experience some scary moments. In those moments, do your best to focus on how scared your loved one must be and stay in the moment with them.

"Kindness can transform someone's dark moment with a blaze of light. You'll never know how much your caring matters."

~ Amy Mercree

A holistic health expert

Be the Patient's Champion

Up until now, we've focused on why it's important to create an army and ways to make that army powerful. This chapter, however, will shift the focus to the patient. After all, supporting someone who is sick is not just about acting as their voice; it's also about showing them love.

I'll share with you how you can further support your loved one and why affection is so important. You'll learn how you can spend quality time with the patient, even if they are bed-ridden. I'll explain why laughter is so important and explore the benefits of palliative care. Last, you'll learn how practicing both compassion and empathy can make a big difference.

AFFECTION

Intuitively, we know that affection can have positive effects on the human psyche. After all, who hasn't had their spirits lifted by a warm hug after a bad day? Humans are hardwired to crave affection.

Kory Floyd, a professor at Arizona State University, studies the connection between interpersonal behavior, physiology, and health. He explains that "skin hunger" is when someone is deprived of meaningful human contact. He has found that people who are deprived of human touch are less happy, lonelier, more depressed, and in worse health than those who receive sufficient physical contact. He concludes that "affectionate contact is so necessary for a healthy life that we suffer when we don't get enough."[6]

It's important to recognize that patients will differ when it comes to the type of affection they prefer. Some will desire hugs and massages while others may only wish to hold hands. If the patient is sedated or in a coma, sensitive touch is still very important.

If you aren't sure what will comfort the patient, it is best to ask them. A Badass Advocate should let the patient know that no request is too big or small. You also may want to offer some suggestions like massaging their hands or feet, rubbing their head, or tickling their arm. No matter what kind of affection you give, be gentle and loving.

I share this information so that you can understand the importance of a loving touch. Seriously ill patients may already feel isolated and lonely. The last thing they should be is deprived of affection.

OWNING CERTAIN RESPONSIBILITIES

When someone is sick, they may not have the energy for certain tasks, such as returning friends' phone calls, paying bills, or tending to their yard. You don't want to encourage a helpless mindset. But you can provide support by accomplishing tasks that aren't critical to getting them back on their feet.

---

[6] https://www.psychologytoday.com/us/blog/affectionado/201308/what-lack-affection-can-do-you

Spending Quality Time

Spending quality time with the patient is one of the best things you can do for them. As mentioned earlier, your loved one may feel lonely and isolated. Just being with them may provide the kind of love and attention they are craving.

First, think of activities the patient enjoyed while they were healthy. Clearly, they probably won't be able to do all of their favorite activities in the same way. For example, strenuous activities like rock climbing are not going to happen. Think of more sedentary activities they may enjoy. While making your list, ask the patient for suggestions.

Here are some other helpful activities that you might consider:

Reading to Them

This can help the patient reconnect with something they enjoyed doing. They may like to hear the sound of your voice and feel comforted that someone is nearby. Plus, it might be more relaxing than watching TV, which can be noisy and irritating.

Soft Music

Playing music quietly can help a patient relax and allow the two of you to enjoy each other's company without feeling the pressure to talk. It also can reduce anxiety, lessen discomfort, and suppress nausea and vomiting.[7]

Music therapy is a growing field that explores how to use music in specific ways to support patients. Music therapists are accomplished musicians who receive training in special techniques that can help

---

[7] https://www.health.harvard.edu/blog/healing-through-music-201511058556

patients relax and even encourage additional healing. If you'd like to find out more, you can find a link to the American Music Therapy Association's website by going to www.badassadvocate.com/resources.

STORY OR JOKE TELLING

Often, Meghan would ask us to tell her stories. I'll be honest: this was challenging for me to do on the fly.

If your loved one enjoys hearing stories from the past, I recommend jotting some down as you think of them. This way, when it's storytelling time, you are prepared and not struggling to come up with one. I especially recommend those stories that can bring about a good belly laugh!

THERAPY DOGS

Many hospitals have therapy dog programs. These dogs can be wonderful for lifting a patient's spirits. My family loves dogs, which meant that *all* of us benefited from their visits.

If the patient has children who love dogs, find out from the nurses when the dogs will be visiting. Try to coordinate it so the children will be present. It is amazing how much joy those sweet dogs can bring. Plus, it makes the patient smile, which is the real goal.

MASSAGE

Massages can be from a professional or a support team member. Keep in mind: you should consult the physician prior to giving any massage to a patient.

Setting the mood is key. You can play some gentle music, dim the lights, and allow the patient to enjoy some quiet, restorative time—which can be especially hard to achieve in the hospital.

GAMES

Playing board games is a great activity for mental stimulation and can be especially helpful for bed-ridden patients. If the patient prefers playing cards, get a magnetic board to prevent the cards from falling to the floor.

LAUGHTER

Laughter is so important that I wanted to highlight it separately.

Lee Berk, an associate professor at Loma Linda University, has spent many years studying laughter's health benefits. He has shown that laughter can cause certain physiological responses like lower blood pressure, lower heart rate, and a stronger immune system.[8]

When it comes to the impact laughter can have on a seriously ill patient, results are inconclusive. However, even if there is no scientific proof that laughter can heal the sick, it certainly can't hurt. At the very least, you can create some new memories that you can cherish for years to come.

> In the summer of 2018, a few of Meghan's very close friends visited her during her long stint in the hospital. At one point, one of her best friends, Julie, came for the weekend. Not only was the visit good for Meghan, but it recharged all of us.

---

[8] https://www.webmd.com/oral-health/video/is-laughter-good-medicine

One night, my brother, Julie, and I decided to sneak some alcohol into Meghan's hospital room. The alcohol was for us, but the mini-party was for Meghan. We wanted to make the most out of our time together.

We spent hours snacking, drinking, telling stories, and laughing. Meghan reveled in it. She wasn't up for a lot of talking back then since it exhausted her. But that night she laid back in her hospital bed and listened to story after story. She giggled the entire night. It was a beautiful memory we all cherish.

For months leading up to that night, life was volatile, terrifying, and depressing like a black, rainy cloud continuously hovered over our family. It had been hard to see the bright side of life.

That night the clouds parted ways, and the sun rays shone through, allowing the four of us to feel genuine joy. For just a few hours, life was as it should be…happy.

Afterwards, the nurses commented on how beneficial laughter can be for a patient. During a dark situation, having a good belly laugh can do wonders.

BE PRESENT

It can be hard for healthy people with busy lives to slow down and spend real quality time with their loved ones. When someone is seriously ill, life begins to resemble a movie. The patient is in slow motion while everyone else is in fast-forward rushing around them. We are so busy trying to manage their illness that we can forget the importance of just stopping to *be* with the actual patient.

Imagine being so sick and lethargic that most of the time you feel alone and isolated. You watch as everyone else's lives go on around you. It's a harsh reality. Being present for the patient is sometimes enough.

The patient may not be up for talking, listening, or playing, and that is okay. Sitting in silence, holding their hand, and loving them is all they may need.

THERAPY

Since this is a difficult time for the patient, they most likely are experiencing a variety of emotions like fear, anxiety, and sadness. They may even be depressed. As a Badass Advocate, it's important to encourage the patient to speak to a professional about their feelings.

After getting their buy-in, you can further support your loved one by setting up a therapy appointment for them. If they are hospitalized, the palliative care team or hospital chaplain can conduct private discussions as well. The goal is to get them talking so they can voice their fears and concerns.

If the patient has young family members, therapy will be important for them as well. Giving young people the space to talk about their feelings may help them cope with the situation better. It's important to speak to children about how therapy can help. There may be free local programs that are specifically designed for their age group.

Unfortunately, many people still view therapy negatively. It may be helpful to consider that most people are not taught how to manage their emotions effectively. This is why patients and their family members may need a neutral party who can teach them this skill.

PALLIATIVE CARE

If your loved one is in the hospital, one resource you can use is the palliative care team. Many people associate palliative care with hospice. But palliative care is much more than end-of-life care. Palliative care is for patients who are seriously ill but not necessarily dying.

A palliative care team consists of doctors, nurses, and other healthcare professionals. They provide patients with continual counseling and support. They focus more on managing the patient's comfort, as opposed to managing the disease. Palliative care also offers programs to support the patient's family and children during this challenging time.

When Meghan was in the hospital, we took advantage of this resource often.

> During Meghan's longer hospitalization, we built a strong bond with one of the palliative care doctors, Dr. Jennifer Aron. Immediately, we recognized Dr. Aron as a kind and gentle physician. Her compassion and professionalism never wavered, even during the most challenging of times.
>
> From the start, it was clear that Dr. Aron's main goal was to improve Meghan's quality of life while in the hospital. She focused on relieving Meghan's physical pain and mental stress. She worked with Meghan on these while her other doctors focused on managing the diseases.
>
> In the end, Dr. Aron's calm and caring nature allowed her and Meghan to build a strong bond. This brought our family great comfort. We knew Meghan trusted Dr. Aron. This relationship gave us peace because we knew that she had a professional to confide in when needed.

Although the focus was on Meghan, Dr. Aron was attentive to the family's needs as well. She consulted us on how to best support Meghan and was open to having honest discussions about her health. The palliative care team also supported Meghan's children during this challenging time.

Dr. Aron even gave me her personal phone number, so we could reach out to her, if needed. I did my best to not take advantage of her good nature. I did, however, text or call her a handful of times when I felt it was truly necessary. There was no limit as to what we could discuss or the support we could request.

What a blessing Dr. Aron and her team were to our family.

If you can find a good palliative care doctor, I highly recommend relying on them for advice and support. After all, the goal of the program is to comfort seriously ill patients and their families.

END-OF-LIFE DISCUSSIONS

Palliative care doctors will champion for the patient in ways the support team may not be able. For example, they can initiate uncomfortable but necessary end-of-life conversations.

Dr. Aron handled many of our more challenging, "what if" discussions. These were topics we dreaded and sometimes avoided. But, Dr. Aron recognized the importance and urgency of these discussions. She unhesitatingly took action and continually comforted us. She assured us that she would own the difficult discussions, so we could focus on loving Meghan.

Her method was to set aside time for private conversations with Meghan in her hospital room. This gave Meghan the opportunity to voice her fears and concerns to a professional.

Dr. Aron also handled conversations about Do Not Resuscitate (DNR) forms. She confirmed what Meghan's desires were if she were to be intubated or fall into a vegetative state. The idea of initiating these types of conversations was heart-wrenching for us. Bringing up end-of-life scenarios felt like we were giving up on Meghan. Giving up was the last thing we were willing to do.

We wanted Meghan to stay in fight mode. On the other hand, we did recognize that she was severely ill, so knowing what she wanted, just in case, was vital.

Dr. Aron started by introducing us to Five Wishes®, which I mentioned earlier. This booklet guides the patient through a difficult but critical decision-making process. It gives the patient five simple and clear key questions to answer.

We would have been fools to not explore advance directives with Meghan. That is why we were so thankful for the work that the palliative care team did. They handled the dirty work while we focused on loving and caring for Meghan. In the end, we didn't need to use the papers that Meghan filled out. But we knew what she truly wanted, which brought us a great deal of comfort.

If these conversations are hard for you to initiate, ask the palliative care team for help. As I mentioned earlier, you can also go to www.badassadvocate.com/resources to find links to Five Wishes® support documents. Remember your goal is to advocate for the patient. Sometimes, advocating means being humble enough to recognize when you can't handle something. When that happens, use the resources that are available to you. Be confident that you are making the right decision by asking a professional for help.

SUPPORT OF CHILDREN

Besides supporting the patient, the palliative care team will also support their children. In a place that can be scary and gloomy for young ones, this can be highly beneficial.

> The palliative care team did a great job of creating positive memories for my young nieces. During hospital visits, Dr. Aron and her team thought of creative ways to entertain them.
>
> Not only did they help make hospital visits more fun, but they improved the quality of those visits, as well. Rather than forcing conversations, they brought activities Meghan and the girls could do *together*. For example, they organized various arts and crafts projects, like thumbprint art or decorating Meghan's hospital room. Decorating the room served two purposes: it was fun for the girls, and it reminded Meghan of the two most important people in her life when they weren't there.

If your sick loved one has young children, I highly recommend asking the palliative care team for ideas. They are experts at making hospital visits more fun and entertaining for kids.

It is challenging to put into words the gratitude I have for the palliative care team, especially Dr. Aron. As I explained, seriously ill patients can benefit significantly from palliative care services. If the patient is terminal, palliative care can help you navigate difficult situations. This is the beauty of the palliative care team. They provide support no matter where the patient is in their health journey.

COMPASSION AND EMPATHY

So far, I have shared some tactical ways to better support the patient during this challenging time. Ultimately, however, what patients need most is compassion and empathy.

Throughout the patient's health journey, the disease will take center stage. Everyone will be working on managing and curing it. This may mean that psychological implications are overlooked. Perhaps compassion and empathy are taking a backseat.

In Christina Feldman and Willem Kuyken's paper, "Compassion in the Landscape of Suffering," they explain that "compassion is a response to suffering, the inevitable adversity all human beings will meet in their lives, whether it is the pain embedded in the fabric of aging, sickness, and death or the psychological and emotional afflictions that debilitate the mind." They go on to say that "compassion is the acknowledgment that not all pain can be 'fixed' or 'solved' but all suffering is made more approachable in a landscape of compassion."[9] This is precisely why showing compassion to a seriously ill patient is so important.

When speaking of empathy, we need to realize that it is not the same as sympathy. As Daniel Pink simply explains in his book *A Whole New Mind*, "Sympathy is feeling *for* another person's pain. Empathy is feeling *with* someone."

Dr. Brené Brown, a researcher who has spent two decades studying empathy, builds on these points. She explains that "empathy requires us to recall or reflect on feelings that are uncomfortable. We're recognizing feelings like frustration, nervousness, or confusion, and trying to take

---

[9] https://pdfs.semanticscholar.org/6e3e/f0f3db6604c1d7e7091e89104b5c56531ba1.pdf

that perspective with another person." Furthermore, she points out that in difficult times "we are hard-wired to need human connection."[10]

To learn more about empathy, I highly recommend checking out Brené Brown's work. She has a video that clearly explains the importance of showing empathy. For me, Brown's insights are both profound and life-changing. I have learned so much from her and believe you can, too. What better time to learn about empathy than now?

BEING EMPATHETIC

If the patient is willing to open up and share how they are feeling, then it's critical that we get our response right. It's normal to feel uncomfortable hearing about the anguish our loved one is in. We want to fix the situation or cheer them up. We need to realize that these reactions won't ease their worries.

In this case, while we are trying our best to be empathetic, we unintentionally fail them. We fail because we don't reassure the patient that we can relate to their pain. Instead, we are trying to put a band-aid on it. The good news is that you can learn how to show empathy.

Professor Theresa Wiseman is a nursing scholar who focuses on both cancer patients' and caregivers' experiences. Her research shows that a big part of the patient experience is receiving empathy. Wiseman has highlighted that, in the eyes of the patient, the difference between an "average" nurse and an "excellent" nurse lies in the nurse's ability to

---

[10] https://twentyonetoys.com/blogs/teaching-empathy/brene-brown-empathy-vs-sympathy

effectively provide empathy, regardless of how that nurse delivers medical care.[11]

If empathy elevates a nurse in the eyes of the patient, imagine how powerful empathy is when it comes from a close friend or family member. Since you are motivated to be an effective caregiver, empathy should be an essential part of your care.

Unsure about how to show empathy? Let's review Wiseman's four attributes of empathy:[12]

1. Putting yourself in someone else's shoes.

2. Avoiding judgment and listening instead.

3. Recognizing emotion in another person that you have maybe felt before.

4. Sharing with that person that you can recognize that emotion.

These four steps will help you to respond in a more empathetic way. With some focus and practice, you can comfort the patient and show them that you accept their feelings about what they are going through.

Next, take your efforts one step further by sharing Wiseman's four attributes with the army. Creating a team of empathetic advocates will significantly help the patient.

---

[11] https://www.researchgate.net/publication/227941757_A_concept_analysis_of_empathy
[12] https://www.habitsforwellbeing.com/the-four-attributes-of-empathy/

UNDERSTANDING THEIR ORDEAL

If you are healthy, then understanding what the patient is experiencing may be a challenge. To better understand their ordeal, you may want to ask the patient to explain it to you. If the patient is not able to explain, then ask the doctor.

I recommend this because of our experience with Meghan. Having a family full of people with healthy lungs, it was hard for us to imagine how her rare lung disease was affecting her. Remember "putting yourself in someone else's shoes" is the first step for expressing empathy.

With all that is going on, you may fail to recognize what the patient is experiencing. If you find that happening, slow down, take a step back, ask questions, and look closely at your loved one's specific experiences and challenges. This will help you shift from a "solving" mindset to an empathetic one.

CONCLUSION

Reading this chapter hopefully gave you some new ideas of how you can advocate for your loved one. On the other hand, you may feel that you are already giving a lot of yourself and don't have the bandwidth to give any more. Giving more to the patient may even feel overwhelming.

First, I don't doubt that you are giving a tremendous amount of your time, effort, and energy to your loved one. Caregiving is a selfless and challenging job.

Second, remember there are many little ways that you can comfort the patient and help them to relax. Not everything has to be grandiose in nature. Just slowing down and spending quality time with your loved one may be all that they need.

Also, let me stress again the first step in becoming a Badass Advocate: build a support team. Caregiving is exhausting, so you need to build your army and then rely on them to do what you cannot. Championing the patient shouldn't fall solely on one person's shoulders. The responsibility is too cumbersome.

Last, don't hesitate to reach out to the palliative care team for that extra boost of help. They are a team of professionals who have the expertise and resources to support you and the patient.

BADASS ADVOCATE ACTIONS:

- ☐ Do not lose sight of the patient. Remember to nurture *their* needs.

- ☐ Make deliberate, continual efforts to spend good quality time with the patient. Knowing you are there for support and fighting alongside them may be all they need to feel at peace.

- ☐ Show loving affection to make a powerful impact.

- ☐ Encourage the patient to see a therapist so they can begin to heal and deal with the severity of the situation.

- ☐ Whether the patient is terminal or not, take advantage of palliative care services. They can support you and your loved one in many ways.

- ☐ Use Theresa Wiseman's four steps to show empathy to the patient.

"There are only four kinds of people in the world. Those who have been caregivers. Those who are currently caregivers. Those who will be caregivers, and those who will need a caregiver."

~ Rosalynn Carter

Former First Lady who founded the Rosalynn Carter Institute for Caregiving, which provides support for caregivers worldwide

Avoid Caregiver Fatigue

So far, this book has focused on the patient and what you can do to powerfully advocate for them. Now, let's switch gears and focus on you, the caregiver. Getting the support you need is essential to your well-being.

Within the healthcare industry, the terms "caregiver fatigue" or "caregiver burnout" are commonly used to describe the serious consequences of caregiving, which can include fatigue, stress, anxiety, and depression. The website www.caregiverfatigue.com clearly explains this phenomenon:

> *Caregiver fatigue primarily refers to the physical exhaustion of looking after a care recipient. However, it is part of a larger descending staircase (metaphorically speaking) where each step leads you closer to caregiver depression. Caregiver stress can be from the physical, mental, emotional, and spiritual toll that the effects of caring for another has upon a caregiver.*

In this chapter, we will focus on how to avoid caregiver fatigue. One important way to avoid it is to implement Badass Strategy #1: create a support team that can help you with the many tasks involved in caregiving.

You'll also need to make time for yourself, even if you think you don't have the time. To stay healthy and strong, you will need to commit to making yourself a priority.

Let me stress the idea of "making time." You deliberately need to take breaks from serving to create your own "soul time"—time that you set aside for activities that bring peace and healing to your heart and mind. "Soul time" does not include running errands or doing housework.

Remind yourself that you are of no good to anyone, especially the patient, if you are worn down. Furthermore, the last thing you want to do is become the patient rather than the caregiver.

VISITATION SCHEDULE

If your loved one needs constant care, one way to make soul time is to create a weekly visitation schedule. If you are the primary caretaker, then you may feel personally responsible for making sure that the patient always has someone by their side. You may feel guilty about leaving the patient. A schedule will give you comfort because you'll know your loved one is being watched over.

Visitors can be spread out to cover time slots that are needed most. Once the schedule is set up, support team members can identify ways to create their own soul time.

Coordinating visitors also ensures that the patient will enjoy a series of fresh and happy (not exhausted) faces. New visitors can share stories, play games, and give updates on what's going on in the outside world. It may be a welcome distraction and could lift your loved one's spirits. Spending time with the patient is also the perfect job for someone who wants to help but doesn't have the time or opportunity to be part of the ongoing care team.

Using an app or website makes it easy to create a schedule. Once the visitation schedule is built, you can share it with friends and family. You can give them access to the scheduling function, if you'd like, and they can choose an open time slot that is convenient for them. If you want a bit more control, you can just assign slots to people on your own and allow them to only "view" the calendar.

Go to www.badassadvocate.com/resources to find links to current websites and apps that can help in setting up visitation schedules.

PATIENT CARE INSTRUCTIONS

The care provided to seriously ill patients can be complicated and restrictive. To help visitors, you can create a patient care instruction sheet.

Imagine being the visitor who is walking into a new situation where the patient's health is at risk. They may be nervous to be left alone with the patient, but at the same time, they desperately want to help. Giving visitors clear directions to follow may calm their nerves and help you to relax too.

The goal of the patient care instruction sheet is to make it as clear and detailed as needed. Include things like directions for medications, patient preferences, and information on when they'll need help. The list could go on, but you get the idea.

Of course, the patient may be able to explain the rules. But re-explaining how things run for every visitor can be exhausting. Furthermore, important details, like when to dose a certain medication, may be forgotten. This can have grave consequences.

An instruction sheet also makes leaving the patient a much smoother transition for the caregiver. Imagine each time you leave having to explain in meticulous detail how to best care for the patient. There are many details you will need to cover so you may not feel comfortable leaving. But if you can hand over a detailed instruction sheet, leaving the patient will be quick and easy.

Last, typing up a set of rules and recommendations gives the visitors confidence. They will know that they can properly support when regular caretakers are absent. No need for them to take notes or remember your directions. You will be organized and have already written out the important details for them.

If you are the primary caretaker, you may not have time to create the patient care instruction sheet. This is a great example of how you can use a support team member to help. Have them create it for you, and you can look it over to ensure nothing is missing.

Good news is I've already created a template for your patient care instructions. To view an example and download a free template, go to www.badassadvocate.com/resources.

HOME HEALTH & HOME CARE

Earlier, I mentioned the possibility of the patient needing constant care at home. Having only one or two people manage at-home care can easily cause caregiver fatigue. One way to manage this ongoing need is to use the services of either a home health or home care company. These companies can support home-bound patients by offering both medical and non-medical assistance.

First, recognize that home health and home care services satisfy different needs.

HOME HEALTH

The first option is home health companies or medical home care. Home health companies offer clinical medical care, performed by licensed nurses, nurse practitioners, and nurse assistants. These services must be prescribed by the patient's physician. If your loved one is hospitalized, home health services may be part of their discharge instructions.

Home health may be covered by insurance, including Medicaid, Medicare, and private insurance. But, there may be limits on the amount of time or visits the insurance company permits. Please do your research if you are interested in home health.

Examples of the services that home health companies can provide are:

- Formally monitoring health status

- Administering of medication

- Injections & changing of IVs

- Wound care

- Vital sign checks

- Consultations on diet & weight

- Physical therapy

- Occupational therapy

- Pain management

- Long-term recovery goals support

- Training on critical care warnings

- Bathing & dressing of patient

If home health support is needed but not prescribed, this is an opportunity for you to be a Badass Advocate. First, set up a meeting with the physician. Then, come prepared with a list of reasons why you believe home health is necessary for the patient's care. Ultimately, it is at the doctor's discretion, but if it is truly needed, they should be easily persuaded.

HOME CARE

The second option is home care companies. These are also known as supportive care, non-medical home care, or private duty. Home care companies offer assistance for activities of daily living (ADLs). Home care is administered by experienced care providers, home health aides, and certified nursing assistants.

While home health may be covered by insurance, home care is typically private pay, meaning it is an out-of-pocket expense. The exception may be when home care is covered by long-term care insurance or Medicaid. If you have set up a donation fund for the patient, paying for home care might be a great use of those funds.

An important tip when hiring a private aide is to validate that they are licensed, insured, and bonded. A licensed aide is properly trained to aid the patient in their day-to-day activities.

Given the access private aides have to a patient's home and possessions, a bonded aide is necessary. If an aide is bonded, it will further protect the patient from theft. When using a personal aide, try to put away credit cards, checkbooks, or other valuables. This isn't to assume all personal aides are thieves, it's just a good idea to take the extra precaution when anyone new comes into the house.

Examples of the services home care companies can provide are:

- Meal preparation

- Light house cleaning

- Laundry

- Bathing, dressing, and grooming assistance

- Companionship

- Transportation (including appointments, events, shopping, and errands)

- Medication reminders

- Incontinence care

- Toileting help

- Ambulation support (reduces risk of falls)

After reading this list, you may feel that you and the support team can handle the home care services. This is probably true. If you can get support team members to own some of these responsibilities, great! However, seriously consider outsourcing these services because they can help prevent caregiver fatigue.

The beauty of hiring a professional is that they can handle the tasks that are sometimes embarrassing for the patient. This is important because it can allow the patient to maintain their dignity. Considering what we know about empathy, you can see how a personal aide can be beneficial.

In summary, here is a comparison of the services that the two types of companies provide:

Service	Home Health	Home Care
Administering of Medications	✓	
Ambulation Support		✓
Bathing & Dressing of Patient	✓	✓
Companionship		✓
Diet & Weight Consultations	✓	
Grooming of Patient		✓
Incontinence Care		✓
Injections & Changing IVs	✓	
Laundry		✓
Light House Cleaning		✓
Long-term Recovery Goals Support	✓	
Meal Preparation		✓
Medication Reminders	✓	✓
Occupational Therapy	✓	
Pain Management	✓	
Physical Therapy	✓	
Toileting Help		✓
Training on Critical Care Warnings	✓	
Transportation		✓
Vital Sign Checks	✓	
Wound Care	✓	

Now identify where you need extra support. Don't let pride and ego get in your way. Be open to receiving the compassionate support you and your loved one need. Recognize that to prevent caregiver fatigue, you must be open to receiving assistance.

MINI-MENTAL VACATIONS

Some days you will be the only one available to support your loved one. In this instance, getting soul time can be challenging, but it is still possible. I recommend a "mini-mental vacation" to, in a sense, get away. If your seriously ill patient tends to sleep often, then that is an opportune time for you to get some soul time. Here are some ideas.

MEDITATION

Clearing your mind through meditation may help you recharge. In fact, transcendental meditation is proven to relieve stress and increase happiness. John Hagelin, Ph.D., scientist, educator, and qualified TM teacher, explains:

> *Happier thoughts lead to essentially a happier biochemistry. A happier, healthier body. Negative thoughts and stress have been shown to seriously degrade the body and the functioning of the brain, because it's our thoughts and emotions that are continuously reassembling, reorganizing, re-creating our body.*[13]

If you have never meditated, there are plenty of quick ways to learn. You can easily find books, apps (e.g. Headspace, Buddhify, Calm), and podcasts that will teach you about meditation. If you want to learn

---

[13] https://thelawofattraction.org/john-hagelin/

more, a simple online search for "meditation" or "mindful meditation" will lead you to a ton of resources.

Now that we have discussed the benefits of meditation, you'll need to find a place to practice. If you are in a hospital, it may be challenging to find a quiet and serene place. Many hospitals do offer a prayer room or chapel where you can meditate (or pray).

Another option may be to find an empty waiting room. I found that some floors in the hospital had very noisy and busy waiting rooms while others were vacant. While the patient is snoozing, go on a little adventure and see what you can find. You can also ask the staff since they probably know which floors or waiting areas tend to be quieter.

Another option is to meditate in the patient's room. While I advocate for getting out of the room, so you can have new scenery, leaving the room may not be an option. When the patient is resting, take advantage of the quiet time.

If the patient is at home, find a quiet room in the house or step outside to breathe in some fresh air. Any place that will allow you some peace and quiet will work.

PRACTICE YOGA

Yoga is exercise that soothes the soul. There are many different types of yoga, so choose one that fits your needs best.

If you are looking for a more relaxing yoga, check out restorative yoga, which is slower paced and uses a series of passive stretches to open up the body. If more movement helps you find inner peace, try hatha yoga.

No matter what kind of yoga you choose, it is a great choice for clearing and calming your mind.

EXERCISE

If exercise is new to you, consult a physician first. Then, find a form of exercise that interests you. If you've tried exercising before and didn't enjoy it or if you feel like you need a change, find a form of exercise that excites you. The goal is to look forward to doing it.

I touched on yoga as one form of exercise, but there are many others that can fuel your body *and* your soul. Running or walking can give you alone time. And alone time is a great opportunity to think through life's biggest challenges.

Other examples to help you get active include: Tai chi, dance lessons, Zumba, rock wall climbing, kayaking, or hiking.

VENTURE OUTSIDE

If your loved one is in the hospital, an easy way to get a mini-mental vacation is to step outside and get some fresh air. I don't know about you, but I never liked the hospital's medicinal smell. Plus, being stuck inside the patient room for hours on end can make you a little stir crazy. Going for an easy stroll while the patient rests may be all that you need to recharge.

During my breaks at the hospital, sometimes I would walk to a local coffee shop, grab a hot drink, and call a friend. The walk outside gave me a break from the room, and the phone call gave me an opportunity to vent.

If I was hungry, I would walk a few blocks further to a cute little café that served delicious, healthy food. The longer walk would give me an extended mental break, and the good food would recharge my body.

If you are a foodie like me, the thought of eating the hospital food may not help your mental state. Do some research! Finding good food within a short distance can give you a chance to get some fresh air *and* lift your spirits.

If there is nothing close, perhaps a food delivery service can bring you some good quality food. Keep in mind, the hospital may not allow outside food in the patient's room. This gives you a great excuse to get out of the room while you eat.

The main point is to try your best to get outside, find some green space, and eat some good food that will support the demands of your caregiver role. Your mind and body will thank you.

READING

If you are sitting with the patient while they are resting, reading can help take your mind off things. Consider books that will help you to escape reality. Don't think about it as avoiding the situation; think of it as giving yourself a reprieve.

WATCH A MOVIE

These days it's easy to watch a movie or miniseries on the go. Streaming services, such as Netflix, HBO Go^{SM}, and Hulu, have apps that allow you to download movies and TV shows directly to your smart device.

If the patient is in the hospital, this is a great way to bring them new content to watch too. It can be challenging to find something enjoyable on the hospital television. If watching on your own, use headphones so you don't annoy or distract others.

JOURNALING

If you've never journaled before, I recommend trying it during this emotional time. Journaling can help you to privately express your thoughts and emotions.

There are many ways to journal, so look for a style or approach that fits your needs. Below are a few ideas to help you get started.

GRATITUDE JOURNAL

A gratitude journal encourages you to take a few minutes to think about what you are thankful for. Of course, it might be challenging to find reasons to be grateful, given your situation. This is understandable. However, I encourage you to keep at it, and come up with at least one small thing.

Don't put the pressure on yourself to think of something profound. You can be thankful for something as minimal as a hot coffee that gives you the extra boost of energy you need. It's not what you are thankful for that is important. It's the act of recognizing that there *are* things for which to be thankful. I promise that creating a habit of being grateful for life, regardless of your hardships, will be worth it.

BRAINSTORMING

During this time, you probably have a lot on your mind. Brainstorming on how to strategize or solve problems may help you to work through those issues.

One great tool to help you brainstorm is mind mapping. Mind mapping can be used on a micro level to solve one specific problem or on a macro level for big-picture strategizing. Below is an example of a macro-level mind map. Keep in mind: there are many ways to mind map, and I am only showing you one.

To create a mind map like the one below, use a piece of paper and pen. It will be easier to quickly jot down ideas as they come to mind. Next, place your main idea or issue in the middle of the page. As ideas begin to flow, continue to branch out from the center, connecting one idea to another.

The goal of mind mapping is to jot down as many ideas as you can until you can't think of any more. Avoid editing yourself. Having an open mind will allow you to think of fresh ideas or come up with more solutions.

Here is an example of a mind map.

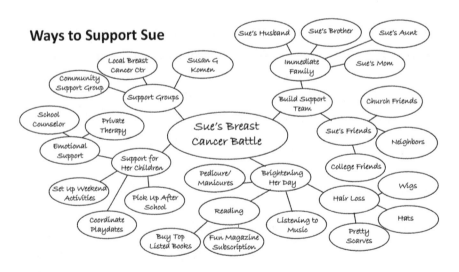

For a free mind mapping template, go to
www.badassadvocate.com/resources.

GOALS & VISIONS

If you don't have one already, you can write down a life vision and yearly goals to help you stay focused and motivated. A vision is the dream you have for your life. Your vision should inspire you. It should get you excited to start the day while you take the steps you need to make that vision a reality.

If you'd like to learn how to create a vision and goals, read Steven Shallenberger's book *Becoming Your Best*. Going through this process can help you clarify what you want out of life. It will help you prioritize your time and stay focused on what is most important.

Furthermore, once you understand how to create a vision and goals, you can teach the patient how to do the same. It may be just what they need to motivate them to keep fighting.

SELF-AFFIRMATIONS

Self-affirmations aren't a form of journaling, but they can be part of your journaling ritual.

Repeating self-affirmations daily is a mental practice that can help you stay focused. Before I began repeating daily self-affirmations, I thought they were foolish. It reminded me of Stuart Smalley from *Saturday Night Live*. The mental image of him looking at his reflection in the mirror and repeating his self-affirmations made it seem ridiculous.

After learning more about the positive impact that self-affirmations can have on the subconscious, I changed my mind. I realized they can help you to stay focused and cultivate a more positive outlook. I learned that many successful people have made self-affirmations a daily practice. If it helps them to stay focused and positive, then it can help you, too.

An example of a good self-affirmation would be:

"I am a Badass Advocate for (patient's name). I do my best to make a difference in her healthcare journey and show her empathy. I am not afraid to ask for help. I continue to practice self-compassion and make self-care a priority."

THANK YOU CARDS

We talked about how being thankful is important for your own mental health. Another way to show gratitude is to thank others for their love and support.

Today, technology makes sending thank yous through email quick and easy. This means, now more than ever, hand-written notes are special and unique. Hand-written notes are appreciated because the recipient knows that these notes take more effort. If you are hanging out while the patient is resting, this is an opportune time to write some thank you cards.

MUSIC

Most of us have experienced how music can impact our souls and can conjure up so many different emotions. It can ignite passion, motivation, and inspiration. It can make you laugh or cry, and it can cause your heart to sing. It can be soothing or moving. During difficult times, music can be a great source of relaxation.

Whatever type of music works for you, tap into this resource. Use music to help you work through the emotions you are experiencing. Looking back, I wish I had turned to music to give me more solace during Meghan's illness.

ART

For some of you, doing art may bring you back to your school days. But using a creative way to express your emotions can help to soothe your soul. You may choose to learn a new skill or practice an old one. Try something like knitting, sewing, painting, drawing, or scrapbooking. Head to a local arts and crafts store and choose something that looks fun!

PUZZLES

Puzzles and word searches can also be a nice distraction. They are good for the brain and help to take your mind off the heavy burdens of life. Head to your local bookstore or search on Amazon to find various types of puzzles and word searches.

IN SUMMARY

There are so many ways that you can take a mini-mental vacation. I gave you some ideas, but you may have some that are more fitting for you. The point is to do what you need, so you can take a brief escape.

THERAPY FOR CAREGIVERS

Don't get me wrong—venting to friends or family can be super helpful, but they aren't professionally trained to guide you through this tumultuous time. Also, they may be closely involved, which means they are dealing with their own stress and anxiety. Expecting to unload on them, on a regular basis, may not be the best idea.

You might have convinced yourself that you are impervious to what is going on. I hate to break it to you, but you aren't. Suppressing or dismissing your emotions will only cause them to show up in other ways.

Working through your emotions is a badass skill. It can help you weather the storm. The best part is that this is a learned skill, and a certified therapist can help. Dealing with a loved one's illness is difficult, and that's why getting a professional to help is imperative.

CHOOSING A THERAPIST

If you haven't met with a therapist before, understand that you may not find the perfect fit immediately. Don't let that deter you. Continue to seek out a therapist that fits you best.

If you are comfortable, I recommend asking friends and family for referrals. Then do your due diligence. Also, check your insurance company's website to find a list of therapists within your network. You might choose using the following criteria:

- Areas of expertise—Check your insurance company or the therapist's website for professional details.

  If your loved one's illness is terminal, you may consider seeking a grief counselor. Even though your loved one is still living, they will have experience in this area. Establishing a relationship early may benefit you down the road.

- Education—You want to be sure the therapist has attended a reputable school. Also, if the therapist attended a college that you have a connection to as well, it may help you to build rapport.

- Designation—Consider what type of therapist is right for you. Below are the differences between the various options:

  Psychiatrists are medical doctors who deal with mental, emotional, and behavioral issues. Since they are doctors, they can prescribe medication. If you feel depressed and think an antidepressant might help, a psychiatrist is a good choice.

  Psychologists have a doctorate in psychology and study the mind and behavior of humans. They cannot prescribe medications, but they can diagnose problems or disorders. They can give you guidance and support throughout your journey.

  Grief Counselors are therapists who specialize in loss, grief, and end-of-life care. Grief counseling can be done either as an individual or in a group.

- Years of Experience—You may want to consider the amount of experience a therapist has under their belt. Whether you chose someone with a lot of experience or not, neither choice is wrong. It's just a preference.

  The therapists I have worked with have had a wide range of experience. The therapist I saw in college was a grad student while the therapist I've seen more recently has over forty years of experience.

  My current therapist gives great life advice, which not all therapists will do. She also has extensive professional and personal life experiences, which she uses to help me through my issues.

- Gender—You may want to see a therapist of the same gender as you. Perhaps you feel more comfortable discussing certain subjects with them. If that's the case, don't feel guilty about that; follow your gut.

Just like all people, therapists come in all shapes and sizes. They can differ in their approach to therapy and in their communication styles. Some will offer advice while others will not. Some will ask a lot of questions while others will let you lead the discussion. All of these approaches are valid; you just need to decide on your preference.

Finding the right fit is sometimes hard. Unless the therapist does something egregious, I recommend attending at least two sessions. Give them a chance before making a final decision. If you find that the second interaction is a negative one, then it may be time to move on.

My overall advice with therapists is to try not to prejudge. If your therapist doesn't look or act like what you imagined, have an open mind. They may surprise you and be exactly what you need.

For therapy to have a fair shot, remember that talking about our emotions is not easy. Some of us are not comfortable sharing emotions with anyone, let alone a stranger. On top of that, talking about such sensitive subjects may make therapy even more difficult to begin. Still, finding space and time to talk about these topics can be very beneficial and help you find more compassion and understanding.

CONCLUSION

Taking care of another human being can be draining. That is why I cannot stress enough the importance of getting additional help. Once you get the help you need, you can take time for yourself. Undertaking the entire responsibility of someone's care is too much for one person to own—even if that someone is your spouse or child.

The point of this chapter is to remind you that you are a priority, too. If you don't take care of yourself, there may be serious consequences, such as caregiver fatigue. Review the self-care ideas I have given you and find intentional ways to give yourself a break.

BADASS ADVOCATE ACTIONS:

- ☐ Set aside soul time for yourself. Participate in activities that bring peace and healing to your heart and mind.

- ☐ Build a visitation schedule so you and the support team can take much-deserved breaks.

- ☐ Consider hiring a professional for medical and non-medical support. To find a reputable company, read reviews, check the Better Business Bureau, and ask healthcare professionals for recommendations.

- ☐ Choose from various mini-mental vacations to reduce stress. Continue to take time for reflection and soothe your soul.

- ☐ Seek out a therapist so you can gain professional advice and get an unbiased opinion.

"Although the days are busy and the workload is always growing, there are still those special moments when someone says or does something and you know you've made a difference in someone's life. That's why I became a nurse."

~ Diane McKenty

Nurse and caregiver

Use the Five Rs Daily

At this point, I've given you seven ways to become a Badass Advocate. All of these are designed to be implemented right away so that you can immediately start providing better care for your loved one—and yourself.

However, becoming a Badass Advocate isn't just about following a sequence of suggestions and then stopping. Instead, it's about following these steps day in, day out so that you can continue to provide the best and most effective care possible without burning out.

Building your team should be your first step, and once you've done that, you won't have to revisit that part of the process every day. But for the remaining Badass Strategies, you'll need to remember to incorporate them into your everyday routine. And this chapter is designed to help you do just that.

FIVE RS

The Five Rs is a 30-minute routine that will help you start the day off strong. Doing it first thing will get you focused before the unpredictability of caretaking monopolizes your day. If you don't have an extra 30 minutes in the morning, you may need to wake up earlier. I promise it will be worth it.

The goal of the Five Rs is threefold. One, it helps you to put the Badass Strategies into practice on a *daily* basis. If you use the Badass Strategies daily, they will eventually become second nature.

Two, the Five Rs will help you stay organized. This should help to decrease anxiety because this 30-minute routine helps you to focus on the most important aspects of caregiving.

Three, the Five Rs will help you to intentionally take a strategic approach to caregiving. You will begin to step out of your comfort zone and go above and beyond to serve the patient. You will act in a respectful manner while acting on the behalf of the patient. You will be determined, persistent, and empathetic. You will create a healthy balance of taking care of the patient while also taking care of yourself. You *will* be a Badass Advocate.

Below are the Five Rs. Feel free to adjust the allotted time based on your own personal needs.

REFLECT (5 MINUTES)

Set aside time to reflect upon your thoughts. You are dealing with a heavy situation. This is the perfect time to write in your journal and repeat your self-affirmations (**Badass Strategy #7**). It is best to start off with **R**eflection to clear your mind and soothe your soul.

1. To assist you in your writing, you can ask yourself questions like:

   - What am I thankful for?

   - What emotions am I dealing with and why?

   - How am I going to face today?

- What is my goal for the day?

- What can I do to keep up my energy?

- When can I set aside a good amount of time (not a short break) for my soul time?

- If I'm not seeing a therapist, should I start?

2. Out loud, repeat your self-affirmation. The one below is an example you can use or use it to help you create your own.

"I am a Badass Advocate for (patient's name). I do my best to make a difference in his healthcare journey and show him empathy. I am not afraid to ask for help. I continue to practice self-compassion and make self-care a priority."

REVIEW (5 MINUTES)

Open the patient's calendar and familiarize yourself with today's schedule. Figure out how the important appointments, meetings, calls, and errands will be completed. Also, you will need to prioritize calling team members whose support you will need that day or week.

When **R**eviewing your calendar, make sure to schedule quality time with the patient (**Badass Strategy #6**) and your daily soul time (**Badass Strategy #7**) for the week. Deliberately enter it into your calendar. Treat soul time and quality time as if they are important appointments that you cannot cancel.

Ask yourself questions like:

- What important appointments/meetings do we need to attend today?

- Who will be driving or attending those appointments/meetings with the patient? *Make a note to remind that person to record the conversation.

- When can I fit in my soul time?

- What do I need to do personally today? When can I accomplish those To-Dos?

- When can someone on the support team have some quality time with the patient today? Does the Director of Delight have something special planned? (suggestions in the Bonus section)

RE-EXAMINE (10 MINUTES)

Start this section by **R**e-examining the patient's care (**Badass Strategy #2**). Once you have purchased a notebook for keeping track of the patient's health information, thumb through it to see if there are any items that need follow-up. If they are not receiving the level of care they deserve, devise a plan to get them what they need.

Also use this time to prepare for any upcoming appointments by organizing the team's list of questions (**Badass Strategy #3**), listening to past recordings (**Badass Strategy #4**), and conducting relevant research (**Badass Strategy #5**).

Re-examine is the longest stage because taking a 10,000-foot view of the patient's case takes time. Some days **R**e-examine will take only a minute while other days it may take over 10 minutes. Budget your time according to what you need to accomplish.

Ask yourself questions like:

- What lingering questions need to be answered?

- How can closed-ended questions be changed into open-ended ones?

- What research needs to be done? Which support team member can take that on?

- Is there a healthcare professional I need to follow up with?

- Is my loved one getting the care they need? If not, what do we need to do to make that happen?

- What future appointments need to be scheduled?

- If there is an item that needs follow up, go back to your calendar. Make sure you set time aside to make it happen or delegate it to someone else.

Re-evaluate (5 minutes)

Take a few minutes to **Re**-evaluate the support team (**Badass Strategy #1**). Are they performing, collaborating, and supporting one another?

Contemplate if someone needs added support. Keep in mind: that someone may be you. Don't be proud! Ask for the help you need and ensure others are getting the support they need, too. Remember this is a team effort.

Ask yourself questions like:

- How am I feeling today? Do I need a break, and if so, who can help?

- Who on the team seems to be struggling? How can we help them?

- When is our next support team meeting? (If you are not the Support Team Leader and no meeting has been set up, they may need a reminder. A simple, gentle reminder should do.)

- Are there any needs that aren't being filled that someone can own?

Once every month or two, you may want to think about the roles everyone plays and if there is a new task someone needs to own.

RECHARGE (5 MINUTES)

Take at least five minutes to meditate (**Badass Strategy #7**). If you feel five minutes isn't enough, I applaud you for taking more time to clear your mind. The goal is to calm your soul before jumping into your day. An easy way to meditate is to find a quiet space, close your eyes, and focus on your breathing.

If meditation isn't your thing, praying or exercising work too. Anything that will help you to feel **R**echarged and ready to face the day! This is your journey so figure out what helps you best.

CONCLUSION

The first few times you do the Five Rs, it may take longer than 30 minutes. Once it becomes a ritual, you will cut down on the time it takes to complete it. Also, don't put pressure on yourself to accomplish everything at once. Remember this is a daily routine, so focus only on the tasks that need your immediate attention. The goal of the Five Rs is to keep you focused on your journey to becoming a Badass Advocate.

Badass Advocate Actions:

☐ **R**eflect—Take time to reflect upon your thoughts and feelings. Show yourself some self-compassion.

☐ **R**eview—Open the patient's calendar and familiarize yourself with the day's schedule. If necessary, remind support team members who need to help that day. Focusing only on that day's plan will help you prepare for what is ahead and reduce feelings of being overwhelmed.

☐ **R**e-examine—Re-examine the patient's care. Reference your notebook and recordings. Determine if any follow up is needed & prepare for upcoming appointments.

☐ **R**e-evaluate—Assess the performance and needs of the support team. Decide if changes need to be made.

☐ **R**echarge—End your Five Rs session with a little self-care. By using something like meditation, prayer, or exercise, you can start your day off strong.

"You gain strength, courage, and confidence by every experience in which you really stop to look fear in the face. You must do the thing which you think you cannot do."

~ Eleanor Roosevelt

Former first lady whose husband was paralyzed from the waist down at 39 years old.

Conclusion

Let me be frank. The situation you are in sucks, but if you are reading this book, it means that you are facing it with courage. It may not feel that way, but you are.

The journey the patient is on can be unpredictable and bumpy. It can include a series of ups and downs, twists and turns. It will refuse to follow a roadmap. You may find yourself heading down a path no one would deliberately choose to take. Nonetheless, you are here, and you need to continue moving forward.

I am so sorry you are going through this challenging time. Unfortunately, nothing anyone says will bring you the kind of comfort you truly need. But you may feel some comfort knowing that you aren't alone.

Each of our situations may differ, but there are so many people in similar situations. That is precisely why I created a private Facebook group called Badass Advocates.

I encourage you to join the group. We are building a network of caregivers to help and encourage one another. You are welcome to come share your story, struggles, or questions.

Self-Compassion

Even if you follow every single one of my suggestions, there still may be times when you are struggling. This is to be expected. At these moments, I encourage you to take a deep breath and be kind to yourself.

Recognize, that being a Badass Advocate is also about taking care of your own mind, body, and soul. Many days you won't feel like much of a badass. Just remember to show yourself some grace. Becoming a Badass Advocate isn't a race but a journey.

Be Proud

Remember to be proud of yourself. You have taken the initiative to be a Badass Advocate, which is not an easy feat. This journey is hard enough, and you are doing the best you can to get your loved one the care they deserve.

You've decided to take charge instead of letting others run the show. After all, you are part of the army that is fighting for someone else's health. Even if the patient doesn't tell you, your determination and commitment bring comfort.

End Self-Doubt

There may be times when you will reflect on what has happened and wonder if you should have made different decisions. You may wonder how another choice would have affected the outcome. Don't do this to yourself. It's counterproductive and a waste of your time.

For those of you whose loved one's illness is terminal, self-doubt is understandable. Although you may not get the happy ending you were hoping for, this situation is not your fault. Remind yourself of that. The little choices you made throughout their health journey would *not* have changed the inevitable. If your loved one dies, it doesn't mean you failed.

If negative, self-doubting thoughts creep in, acknowledge them, and remind yourself that you are doing the best you can during this challenging time. Give yourself the gift of self-compassion. Focus on your valiant efforts and time well spent with your loved one.

FORGE FORWARD

At the end of each day, focus on moving forward. Recognize that you are doing your best to support your loved one. Immediately start implementing the Five Rs. Once you begin to put the Badass Strategies into place, you will begin to see the difference you can make.

Remember, the most important act of a Badass Advocate is to be present. You want your loved one to know they have an army of advocates fighting alongside them. Follow the eight Badass Strategies and you *will* be the champion your seriously ill loved one deserves.

Good luck in your journey!

Bonus
Assemble Your Care Team

Support Team Roles

To help you set up your army of advocates, I am listing out some ideas for possible roles. Everyone's situation is different, so while some of these roles may be a great fit, others won't make sense for your situation. You don't have to follow the roles exactly. You can cherry-pick the ideas that work best for you and the patient.

For Meghan's support team the roles weren't as clearly defined. We didn't go in with a plan because we didn't have anyone to show us the way. We were figuring it out on the fly. That is why I wrote this book, so you can learn from us and do better than we did.

You also don't need a ton of people on your support team. If you have a hard time finding people to join the team ask a few kind souls to own some of the smaller, less important tasks. This alone can greatly alleviate some of your stress.

Many caregivers feel that they must take on everything by themselves. Although much of the actual caring of the patient may fall on one person's shoulders, good friends and family members can still provide meaningful help. For example, you could have a young, trustworthy cousin handle the donation fund. Or you could have a rotation of good friends visit once a week to lighten the patient's spirits.

Get creative and realize that you don't have to go it alone. Be open to receiving help. Read on for some ideas as to how you can get others to chip in!

"Caregiving often calls us to lean into love we didn't know possible."

~ *Tia Walker*

Author who wrote a book called The Inspired Caregiver, which focuses on the unsung hero, the caregiver.

CARE COORDINATOR

The Care Coordinator is the most important role on the support team. This responsibility will most likely fall onto someone like a spouse, parent, or adult child. This person handles the management, organization, and coordination of the patient's care. Below I will explain why this role is critical and the responsibilities that might be part of this role.

ELECTRONIC MEDICAL RECORDS

Since the early 2000s, the US healthcare system has been converting paper charts to electronic medical records (EMRs). An EMR is a digital version of a patient's paper medical chart. The implementation of EMRs has made a considerable impact on the coordination of patient care, allowing providers to integrate medical records, record treatment plans, and manage drug information.

You may find that some health systems are further along in the process of switching over to EMRs. And the more integrated the health system, the easier it is for providers to share medical information.

EMRs may streamline the sharing of patient information, but the need for coordination of care still exists. Because physicians do not own the coordination of care, a Care Coordinator is needed.

Remember physicians have many patients they are taking care of, while your badass team has one. They are the healthcare *provider* while you are the patient's *advocate*. This doesn't mean that physicians don't advocate for their patients, because they do. It means that advocates are focused primarily on advocating while physicians are primarily focused on providing good care.

The Care Coordinator doesn't need a medical degree to do a good job. Rather, their job is to pay close attention, ask questions, and speak up when something seems off.

COORDINATION OF CARE

The need for a Care Coordinator becomes especially important when a patient is being treated by several providers. In this case, this person will need to "manage" the coordination of the patient's care. They may need to find the right doctors, set up appointments, submit insurance claims, and so on.

The lack of coordinated care within the healthcare system is why this role is so important. I'll warn you that taking on this role can be a significant challenge. But giving a patient this high level of support is critical to optimizing care.

> As you know, my sister was dealing with three diseases concomitantly. She had an autoimmune disease, cancer, and a lung disease. Having three diseases meant she was being evaluated by three specialists, including an oncologist, pulmonologist, and oral surgeon. On top of those providers, she also had a physical therapist and home health nurse helping her.

Early on, we realized that one provider wouldn't be overseeing her entire case. Instead, we needed a hub in the middle of what had become a multi-spoke treatment regimen. Our mom, who is retired and a natural nurturer, became Meghan's Care Coordinator. This is how she describes the role:

I was coordinating doctor appointments, home nurses, PT, and more. I kept a journal, which was so important because it allowed me to keep it all straight. It's all so overwhelming. On top of that, you are caring for someone you love, which makes it hard to keep your head straight. Care Coordinators feel responsible for everything. The patient needs to concentrate on their treatment, how they feel, and getting better. The patient's well-being weighs heavily on the caregiver's mind and heart.

CARE COORDINATOR'S RESPONSIBILITIES

The Care Coordinator's responsibilities may include:

- Scheduling, coordinating, and attending doctors' appointments.

- Preparing for upcoming appointments.

- Ensuring that conversations with the doctor are recorded and shared with the team.

- Keeping track of the patient's health information.

- Paying close attention to details and taking diligent notes.

- Booking appointments with new healthcare professionals. The patient may need a nutritionist, physical therapist, or psychologist.

Since the Care Coordinator has many responsibilities, there may be times when other team members need to step up and help. They can support by taking the patient to doctor's appointments, picking up medications, and so on. I highly recommend having a list of back-up helpers the Care Coordinator can rely on in case they need assistance with one of these key responsibilities. Delegating may reduce stress on overwhelming days. By creating a strong support team, the Care Coordinator won't have to carry the entire burden of care.

If your loved one is hospitalized, there are many ways the Care Coordinator can advocate for the patient. For example, shift changes tend to be a chaotic time. The staff will be in the process of sharing patient information. Yet, a well-informed Care Coordinator can support them during this time by giving patient updates. They also can catch mistakes, if they happen.

Having a Care Coordinator is important because they know the patient personally. The nurse who is taking over may have a question after the previous nurse has left. If the Care Coordinator is there, they can support the new nurse. These are just a few important ways the Care Coordinator can benefit the patient while hospitalized.

HOSPITAL CASE MANAGER

If your loved one is hospitalized, they will be assigned a hospital case manager who is responsible for managing their care. This person is typically a nurse, though not the head nurse, which is a different role.

The hospital case manager will coordinate care among hospital staff, including doctors, physical therapists, and dietitians. They will also organize the patient's discharge and transition the patient to post-care. You may rarely see this person since they act on behalf of the patient in the background.

If your loved one is in the hospital for a longer stay, get the case manager's information. Building a relationship with this person will allow the Care Coordinator to stay informed. If there are questions the staff cannot answer about the patient's care, ask the case manager.

My mom would reach out to the hospital case manager to ask questions and understand the next steps. Being informed meant we could better advocate for Meghan while she was in the hospital.

If the Care Coordinator gets the case manager's information, they should not abuse this privilege. Rather, they should contact them only when they really need information. If the Care Coordinator is uncomfortable reaching out, they must remind themselves that this is what it takes to be a Badass Advocate. Remember, their actions are on the behalf of someone who cannot do it for themselves.

PROFESSIONAL PATIENT ADVOCATE

At this point, it is important to make you aware of the professional designation of patient advocate. A patient advocate can help patients to navigate the healthcare system. Hiring a healthcare expert to act on the patient's behalf can be very beneficial.

A patient advocate might attend doctor's appointments, consult with providers, help the patient make decisions, and also decipher and dispute insurance bills. They can even help the patient find legal or financial advice.

Hiring a patient advocate doesn't completely eliminate the need for a Care Coordinator. A patient advocate can, however, be a beneficial resource.

If you are interested in hiring a patient advocate, I recommend asking for a doctor referral. You can also use the internet to find many companies that offer these services. To find someone reputable, be diligent in your research. Also, if your loved one is hospitalized, they may have one on staff that you can use.

Now let's dive into how to powerfully own the role of Care Coordinator.

CARE COORDINATOR QUALITIES

The Care Coordinator needs to be well-organized, assertive, focused, and diplomatic. Since you are the one reading this book, this role may naturally fall on your shoulders. If that is the case, then you'll need to remind yourself that everything you do is on behalf of the patient. To be a badass Care Coordinator, you'll need to pay close attention and speak up when necessary.

If this role falls on someone else, like a significant other, parent, or sibling, you may need to lend a hand. If they are disorganized or apprehensive, figure out ways to fill in the gaps. Mistakes can happen, so having a strong voice is important. This means someone must pay close attention to detail and address any issues.

ORGANIZATION

The first task as a Care Coordinator is to get organized. They will receive a barrage of information, so keeping track of it from day one is imperative.

As a Care Coordinator, one of their most important roles is to take and keep diligent notes. If they haven't already, they will need to buy a fresh notebook and use it only for the patient's care. If they prefer to go paperless, there are many note-taking apps available.

Below is some information they will want to keep track of in the notebook:

- Doctors' names & contact information

- List of medications (including frequency and dose) and allergies

- List of diagnoses and prognoses (including official disease names)

- Topline instructions from providers (reference audio recordings and other team member's notes)

A well-organized notebook is important for the following reasons:

- Notes will help them to stay focused and prevent misinformation.

- Physicians may conflict on subjects like diet, exercise, and treatment. Having detailed notes will allow the Care Coordinator to follow up and clarify the next steps.

- A notebook will help the Care Coordinator keep track of questions so that they can reference them on future visits.

- It's imperative to track key points each physician shares. The Care Coordinator may need to go back and listen to recordings (Badass Strategy #4) to make sure they haven't missed anything. Bullet point the items in the notebook, so they are easy to reference.

- The Care Coordinator may need to relay information back to physicians who don't have hospital privileges. It's important to keep everyone aligned.

They'll also need to buy a new calendar or use a digital one. One benefit of a digital calendar is that they can easily share it with the support team. This streamlines communication and allows them to better coordinate schedules.

BADASS CARE COORDINATOR ACTIONS:

☐ Get organized by using a notebook or app to record specifics about the patient's health.

☐ Buy a calendar or use a digital one to stay on top of the patient's appointments, meetings, etc.

☐ Be diligent in taking note of details pertaining to the patient's care.

☐ When in the hospital, build a relationship with the hospital case manager. They are a great resource and can keep you informed on the patient's case.

☐ Be open to relying on others for support and don't hesitate to ask for help.

♡

"Helping others isn't a chore; it is one of the greatest gifts there is."

~Liya Kebede

A WHO Goodwill Ambassador who founded the Liya Kebede Foundation. The foundation's mission is to reduce maternal, newborn, and child mortality in Ethiopia and around the world.

Support Team Leader

The Support Team Leader will be responsible for organizing, coordinating, and managing the group. They help the team to stay aligned and work together. The idea of organizing a team may seem unnecessary, but the more organized you are, the more badass you will be.

One duty of the Support Team Leader will be to assign each team member a role. While assigning roles, it will be imperative to avoid being a dictator. No adult wants to be told what they *have* to do without having their opinion heard. People can become resentful if they're given a role they don't want or if they feel like their input is ignored. That can cause more issues and headaches for you in the long run.

Remember: this isn't a team of professionals at work; this is a team of friends and family who are volunteering. Out of the goodness of their hearts, these individuals want to help the same sick person you do. The Support Team Leader's focus should be to keep this group of individuals connected and collaborating.

Choosing Roles

After the Support Team Leader decides on who will be a part of the team and which roles are needed, they will need to work with the team members to decide on who is best for each role. Below are suggestions for how to decide who should take on which team role.

IDENTIFY STRENGTHS & KNOWLEDGE

Recognize others' strengths and knowledge. Then, capitalize on them.

There are many talents you can use to help the patient. For instance, if someone in the group is a great cook, suggest that they take on the role of the Meal Train Organizer. They can cook some of the meals, gauge when meals are needed, and give donors suggestions.

This is only one example of how others' strengths can benefit the patient. Take into consideration others' knowledge, capabilities, and living distance to the patient. You may be surprised at how others' strengths can come in handy.

Furthermore, if there are areas of care you need help with, consider who has knowledge in that area. There are many areas of expertise that can help the group. Brainstorm with the group so you uncover all opportunities. Then tap into your resources to build a badass army.

LEVERAGE PAST EXPERIENCE

Don't underestimate the value of having someone on the team who has been a caregiver in the past. As unfortunate as it was, my family was able to better support Meghan because we had been through it with our dad. We learned from our past and used that knowledge to our advantage. If you are new to caregiving, I highly recommend leaning on others who have been caregivers before.

Use Connections

Consider the connections support team members may have within the community. Then, strategize on how those connections may benefit the patient.

If you feel uncomfortable doing this, remind yourself that to be a Badass Advocate you need to take action. Badass Advocates aren't afraid to leverage connections to influence the patient's care.

Consider Location

Take into consideration where team members live. If some team members don't live close by, that may affect what roles they can take on, but they can still help the patient and the family in significant ways.

Support Team Leader's Responsibilities

Now that The Support Team Leader understands what to consider when assigning roles, let's talk about their responsibilities. When it comes to managing the team's roles, the Support Team Leader has three main goals:

1.Re-evaluate Roles—Check in with team members every so often to see how they are handling their role. If their role is challenging, they may find they can't manage the role as well as they had originally thought. The solution may be as simple as needing a change or some extra support.

While brainstorming solutions, always take into consideration what's best for the patient. Below are some ideas that may help:

- Pair up team members—Ask a few support team members to work together in the same role. They can alternate days and times so the others can have a break. It may be best to create a weekly schedule, so expectations are clear. This way, the burden won't fall on one person's shoulders.

- Take advantage of non-support team members—At times, your army of advocates may not be enough. If that is the case, tap into other resources like those who have been asking how they can help.

  Non-support team members can always take on smaller or less significant tasks. For example, one support team member may be responsible for managing the patient's house. In this case, ask someone who is wanting to help to walk the dog or unload the dishwasher. They are small jobs that can be a huge help.

- Hire a professional—You can hire out almost anything these days. Meaning, there are various professionals who can help lessen your load. Consider hiring a private chef, cleaning service, dog walker, or babysitter. If you can afford to pay for someone to take over small tasks, this is a great way to reduce some stress.

Let me share an example.

During the summer of 2018, Meghan had a long stint in the hospital. When she got home, she still needed assistance walking to the bathroom. We could easily help her during the day, but the middle of the night runs were becoming challenging. Sleeping on a chair next to her every night became increasingly difficult for our family.

As a solution, her husband hired a night nurse. This allowed worn-down family members to get a good night's rest, so they could perform their duties the next day, and Meghan received some much-needed support throughout the night. This solution significantly reduced the stress put on our family.

I realize everyone may not have the financial means to pay out-of-pocket for added support. If that is the case for you, be sure to check the patient's insurance company for more details on covered services.

If you haven't already, make sure you read the section under Badass Strategy #7 on home health and home care. You will gain a better understanding of what these are and what services they offer.

2.Accountability – If a support team member isn't living up to expectations, you will need to address the issue. Talk to the team member compassionately in order to better understand what is going on and to review expectations.

During the discussion, focus on being empathetic. A loved one's illness can take a toll on anyone involved. First, aim to understand their perspective before jumping to conclusions. You may be making the wrong assumptions. Using your listening skills will help. Try to be as gentle as possible and remind them how important their role is and how it helps the patient.

That conversation might sound something like this:

> *Tom, I wanted to touch base with you about being Sarah's Meal Train Organizer. Catch me up on what's been happening with the meal train program.*
>
> *(Listen intently as he gives you his perspective. If something isn't clear, continue to ask questions. Your goal is to better understand why he isn't*

living up to the role's expectations. If he no longer wants the job, he may hint at needing help or a replacement before you need to suggest it).

I hear what you are saying. This job may be more work than what we first anticipated. I know Sarah and her family appreciate what you've done so far. Without the food donations, Sarah might not get the healthy meals she needs to build her strength. Plus, her husband, Bill, wouldn't get a break from cooking dinner every night for the kids.

It's important that as her support team we make this process as easy as possible for those who wish to help. You mentioned you haven't set up an app yet. When were you planning on setting that up? Would it be helpful if I ask someone else on the team to take that on? The meals are super important, so I want to be sure it is done in the next day or two so those who want to help can. Let's brainstorm on how we can make that happen.

Going forward, I want to be sure you still want to take on the role of Meal Train Organizer. I understand if you have too much on your plate right now. I only ask because I want to ensure Sarah and her family are getting everything they need. It's important we have someone take full ownership of organizing the meals.

How do you feel about it? Are you still interested in organizing the meal train, or would you like me to find someone else to own this role? There are no hard feelings if you want to graciously bow out.

The goal of the conversation is to be empathetic while communicating the seriousness of the role. You will need to review expectations and then ask for a renewed commitment.

3.Encouragement – Being a caretaker is a thankless job. Rightly so, the patient needs all the love and attention they can get. However, this means those who are sacrificing a lot may feel underappreciated.

It may be a good idea to give one another pats on the back during team meetings or on your group chats. Telling others what a great job they are doing may encourage them and give them the boost they need.

Since you are the one taking charge, I'm hoping that you too will get some recognition and encouragement. Share the idea of encouragement with the group so you can support one another. The Director of Delight (discussed in a later chapter) may have a creative way to celebrate the team.

MEETINGS

Once the Support Team Leader has the support team in place, they will need to set up a regular group meeting. For each meeting, they should create an agenda. An agenda will help the team to stay on task. The Support Team Leader should also survey team members to see if other subjects need to be covered.

Topics of discussion may include:

- Organization of and updates on medications

- Hospital visitation schedule

- Upcoming doctors' appointments

- Patient's child care coordination

- Management of donations

- Patient's financial situation (may not be an appropriate subject to discuss depending on the team)

- Insurance concerns or questions

- Updated information from physicians/hospital

There may also be topics specific to your team dynamic and loved one's situation. Team meetings allow everyone to be on the same page, voice concerns, and ask questions.

CONCLUSION

The main goal of the Support Team Leader is to minimize stress by keeping the team aligned. Having each member clear on their role will promote cohesiveness and teamwork. After all, taking care of a sick loved one is hard to do on your own. Building a support team where everyone knows their role will help reduce stress.

Ultimately, the Support Team Leader should tailor each team member's role to fit the patient's needs. Feel free to add and eliminate as needed, based on the patient's situation. The roles I list in this book are just ideas to help your team get started. The titles aren't important either. They are silly names I used to make it light-hearted.

In the end, the Support Team Leader will want to gain agreement from everyone that they are comfortable with their role. Checking in during face-to-face meetings is a good time to reassess. The Support Team Leader can ensure team members are happy in their role and getting the additional support they need.

BADASS SUPPORT TEAM LEADER ACTIONS:

☐ Create and assign customized roles by working with each team member. Be sure to consider each person's strengths, experiences, expertise, connections, and availability.

☐ Periodically re-evaluate team roles. You'll want to ensure members are satisfied with their role and willing to carry on with their duties.

☐ Keep the team's line of communication open by creating a forum for the group to chat.

☐ When holding team members accountable, be gentle yet stern. Remember their level of dedication and participation directly affects the patient. Address issues promptly and tactfully.

☐ Set up your first team meeting. Then, set the precedent that support team meetings will be a regular occurrence. The frequency of meetings will depend upon the needs of the team and the patient.

☐ Schedule regular team meetings so the group stays connected and aligned with the total care of the patient. Come to each meeting with an agenda and topics that need to be addressed.

☐ Celebrate team members and their hard work so they know they are appreciated.

♡

"The aim of medicine is to prevent disease and prolong life, the ideal of medicine is to eliminate the need of a physician."

~ William J. Mayo

A physician and surgeon who was one of the seven founders of the Mayo Clinic

Master of Medications

One way to reduce medication mistakes is to have a Master of Medications who learns about and manages each medication. This is especially important when your loved one is taking many medications.

Master of Medications' Responsibilities

Learning about medications may take time, and each medication will serve a different purpose. Dosing schedules can be inconsistent, and instructions can be complicated. This may be overwhelming and confusing for the patient. Understanding what each medication does is a big part of being a Badass Advocate.

If possible, the patient should be knowledgeable about the meds they take. When they are coherent, they should take charge of administering their own meds. If they tend to already be confused, allowing them to be in charge of their meds is a big risk.

This is why it is important to identify a team member to learn about the medications and the schedule.

> Meghan's medications could become overwhelming because there were a lot of them. On top of the amount she was taking, the medications were administered at varying times. Some were dosed every six hours while others were dosed

every eight or 12. Keeping it straight was important but challenging.

That's when I came up with the idea of creating a spreadsheet to help us make sure she didn't miss a dose. The spreadsheet included specifics about each medication. It listed each medication's name, milligram strength, and prescribed dosing. We would then mark down the time she took each medication. The spreadsheet helped us to monitor her progress.

If the Master of Medications would like a blank copy of the spreadsheet I created, they can download a free version at www.badassadvocate. com/resources. Once they download the spreadsheet, they can edit it and make it their own.

If creating their own spreadsheet is too cumbersome, they should consider using an app. There are many medication tracking apps available, like Medisafe Medication and Round Health. These apps are not as customizable, but they can help you to organize the patient's medication schedule. Another benefit is that an app allows the patient to easily track their own medication schedule from their phone.

Be Knowledgeable

A serious disease can make managing medications overwhelming and confusing for anyone. On top of that, medications may cause the patient to become unfocused and fuzzy. A confused patient can easily make a mistake. The patient may accidentally skip, underdose, or overdose their medications. This is why having an advocate to help manage their medications is imperative.

A medication tracker will also come in handy during an emergency. Medical staff will need a list of medications. During this critical time, you don't want to rely on the patient to relay this information.

In fact, having several team members familiar with the medications is highly beneficial. That is because there will be times when the Master of Medications won't be available. For example, they may need to travel, have a night off, go to work or school, or run errands. If there is no one to fill in, this can leave the patient in a bind. Having a replacement is imperative.

Those who will be managing medications should be reliable, organized, detail-oriented, and intelligent. They will need to know key information about each medication, like indications, usage, dosage, administration, possible contraindications, and side effects. This information can be found in the medication's patient package insert (PPI), a document that comes with prescription medication and instructs patients on how to safely use the medication.

Because a PPI contains FDA-approved labeling, it is more reliable than finding information about a product via a Google search. The Master of Medications should be wary of what they find online as this information may be skewed. Their best bet is to call the prescribing doctor's office if they have any questions or concerns.

CONCLUSION

I realize the Care Coordinator may be the person to also own the Master of Medications role. In many cases, owning both roles makes the most sense. However, owning the two roles with the most responsibility is a lot to handle.

Do your best to teach others how to manage some of the tasks, so they can step in when necessary. Sharing this responsibility with others will give you the freedom you will need.

The Master of Medications is a serious role. Medication errors are common, so those responsible for managing drugs need to pay close attention. Being aware of the risks and staying organized should help minimize mistakes.

BADASS MASTER OF MEDICATIONS ACTIONS:

- ☐ Get organized by either using a medication tracking spreadsheet or an app. You can access a free downloadable medication tracker at www.badassadvocate.com/resources.

- ☐ Familiarize yourself with the patient's medications (medication name, what it treats, dosing, mg strength, warnings, contra-indications, etc.). The more familiar you are with the medications, the better you can support.

- ☐ Train other support team members on the patient's medications and medication tracker. This is especially important if the meds are complicated. Having a back-up partner will alleviate some pressure and stress.

- ☐ Keep the medication tracker current so the patient isn't overdosed or missing doses.

"It's not how much we give, but how much love we put into giving."

~ *Mother Theresa*

A humanitarian who continually found ways to advocate, provide care and give peace to the sick and dying.

DONATIONS MANAGER

Raising funds can be a great way to support the patient and their family. It can help pay for healthcare expenses, unforeseen personal needs, and more. The Donations Manager will need to be trustworthy, organized, and ethical. If you plan to set up a fund-raising website, also known as crowdfunding, being tech savvy is also important. Visit www.badassadvocate.com/resources for a list of crowdfunding websites.

If the Donations Manager lives in the same house as the patient, it may be better etiquette to have someone else set up the donation fund. Sometimes when those who live with the patient ask for donations, it may sound like they are asking for handouts. On the other hand, when someone else asks for donations, it feels more like they are doing a good deed.

DONATIONS MANAGER'S RESPONSIBILITIES

One key role of the Donations Manager is to organize and manage the donations. Management of donations is especially critical when they are desperately needed or overflowing.

> During Meghan's illness, we had many generous people offer their support to Meghan and her family. She had a continuous flow of meals, gifts, and sweet treats. It was incredible. We

were all so thankful for people's thoughtfulness and generosity.

After a while, my sister's house was overflowing with meals and her family couldn't consume them all. Don't get me wrong: we were thankful for every single donation. At the same time, we wanted to make the most out of people's kindness. Our goal was to redirect the donations from food to other necessities.

If we had monetary donations, we could cover some unexpected costs that recently popped up. It was time to begin managing the influx of donations.

CROWDFUNDING

Based on my experience, I highly recommend setting up a crowdfunding account. A crowdfunding site will help you to more easily and efficiently manage the monetary donations.

Remember that the importance of accepting monetary donations is to fit them to the needs of your loved one. Patient needs may include:

- Out-of-pocket medication costs

- Hospital charges

- Medical equipment

- Physical therapy

- Private nurse

- Private chef (for extremely strict dietary needs)

No matter how you set up the donation fund, the person in charge needs to be trustworthy and ethical. People will want to know that 100% of their donations will go to helping the patient.

ACCEPTING HELP

If the patient is not struggling financially, asking for donations may be uncomfortable. However, asking for or receiving help in a time of need doesn't make them selfish or greedy. During difficult times, they will need to be open to accepting help.

Accepting help and compassion can be challenging for many of us. However, a 2013 study in the journal *Mindfulness* focused on the connection between practicing self-compassion and receiving compassion. It notes that "social support in times of distress helps us cope with and recover from life's difficult moments."[14] Do not think of accepting help as weakness, but as an opportunity to heal and grow.

Also, even if your loved one is fortunate financially, keep in mind there may be unforeseen costs in the future. Organizing donations may help to mitigate financial stress. If the Donations Manager feels uncomfortable accepting donations, remind them that their actions are on behalf of the patient. Badass Advocates form armies to back up the patient, and this is one way to build your army.

I'll share how I handled asking for donations in hopes that it gives you some ideas. Pay attention to the transparency in my communication. Being honest and open is the best way to ask for help.

---

[14] https://www.researchgate.net/publication/319243762_Practicing_Self-Compassion_Weakens_the_Relationship_Between_Fear_of_Receiving_Compassion_and_the_Desire_to_Conceal_Negative_Experiences_from_Others
https://greatergood.berkeley.edu/article/item/how_to_open_yourself_up_to_receiving_help

For people who *wanted* to help but weren't sure *how*, I typed up a text message to explain how they could support Meghan. I wrote something like:

Dear Friends and Family,

As all of you know, Meghan was diagnosed with non-Hodgkin's lymphoma on Sept. 13th, 2017. Some of you are also aware that she has an autoimmune disease, which has caused her to drastically change her diet and lose weight. Many of you have asked what you can do to help.

We do not have an official Go Fund Me page but are taking donations to help defray costs for a private chef who will take care of Meghan's meals, medical expenses not covered by Meghan's insurance, and a private nurse who we are hiring to help with home infusions. They need to be administered two and three times a day through January. We are accepting donations via Venmo, or you can mail them to…

Donors could send a check or Venmo me, and I would deposit them into an account for Meghan and her family. We immediately began to receive donations. Easy as that.

A few months later, the funds began to dwindle due to Meghan's new diagnosis of BO and the rising healthcare costs that accompanied it. It was time to send a reminder text message. Once again, the donations started rolling in. Throughout the year, we raised over $20,000 from just two requests. Keep in mind, we have a large loving family and Meghan has a lot of generous friends.

These funds meant that Meghan didn't have to stress about paying for some unforeseen expenses. We were able to give Meghan the extra care that she needed without financial worries.

The process of collecting donations was simple and straight-forward. It worked well for our family. If necessary, I hope it does for yours, too. Like I said, I would recommend using a crowdfunding site. It is much easier to manage than collecting and depositing checks.

RECEIVING GIFTS

There may be people who would rather give an actual present than money. That's okay, too. Gifts can be more sentimental and personal. Any generosity should be welcomed.

For some unique gift ideas go to www.badassadvocate.com/shop.

If you want to search for your own gift, below are some ideas to get you started.

HOME-COOKED MEALS

Donating meals may be obvious and most will think of it on their own. Yet, you can only eat so much pasta, right? If people are asking to donate meals, refer to the next chapter. In it, we will discuss the role of Meal Train Organizer and how they can organize donated meals.

BLANKETS

If your loved one has lost weight or is going through chemo, they may tend to be cold a lot. Blankets are a great gift and having more than one is never a bad idea. One can be placed in their hospital bag while others can be positioned around the house for easy access. The big, soft ones are the best, and you can find them in all sorts of price ranges.

If donors are crafty, they can take it one step further and make a blanket like the one my sister's dear friend, Kate, did. It was heavy, soft, and made from the heart. Considering it was handmade from a friend, it ended up being my sister's favorite. It constantly traveled to and from the hospital with her.

HATS/SCARVES

For patients who will lose their hair, hats and scarves can be a nice supportive gift. Consider their style and what they would enjoy wearing.

NON-SLIP SOFT SOCKS/SLIPPERS

Patients who are frail and thin may have cold feet. Super-soft socks are a great gift for someone who is couch-bound or bedridden. If your loved one is fragile, grippers will be necessary to help prevent falls.

COZY WRAP

Again, if the patient tends to be cold, having something warm to wrap up in is a thoughtful gift. If the patient is connected to monitors or has a hard time lifting their arms, a wrap may be most appropriate.

OVERNIGHT BAG

If your loved one is traveling back and forth to the hospital, a nice travel bag is a good idea. I recommend a bag that has wheels, good storage, and several compartments.

The most important feature to consider is size. The bag should be large enough to hold a few days' worth of clothes, as well as favorite items from home like a blanket or stuffed animal. One of my favorite companies is Mark & Graham®. They have nice looking personalized, leather bags.

MAGAZINES

Television can get mundane after a while, and the patient may be irritated by the noise. Magazines are easy, quick reads and don't take a long-term commitment. Find what interests the patient and buy a magazine or a subscription about this subject. Reading also helps to keep their mind sharp.

BOOKS

Books are a longer commitment. But if the patient is coherent and likes to read, finding a fun or interesting book to read may help them relax.

LOTION/CREAM

Certain medications may dry out the patient's skin. Giving a high-quality lotion or cream may be a nice treat. I recommend looking for ones with fewer chemicals and more natural ingredients.

OVERWHELMED WITH GIFTS

If the patient receives a barrage of people offering gifts, I'm thrilled for you! Be thankful you have so many kind souls in your life.

If the number of offers is overwhelming, don't be embarrassed to say, "I appreciate your offer. You have no idea how much it means to us. Luckily, we don't need X right now, but we did set up a donation fund to pay for unforeseen costs. If you are interested in contributing, I'm happy to send you more information."

Clearly, you don't want to turn away someone who is standing at your door with a container of hot lasagna. Use this line with someone who is preemptively offering to donate something you don't need. This approach will give the donor an out. At the same time, if they decide to give, they can help in a more productive way. I found that most people were happy to get a recommendation because they truly needed one.

Conclusion

The Donations Manager must consult the patient to ensure all funds are properly allocated. First, they should gain an understanding as to how much the monetary goal is, and then aim to reach it by sending out regular reminders. Once the donation fund hits the goal, the Donations Manager and patient must use the money as promised.

Remember the goal is to be a Badass Donations Manager, which means their actions should always be for the good of the patient. Dr. Brené Brown says it best in her book *The Gifts of Imperfection* when she writes:

> *"Somehow we've come to equate success with not needing anyone. Many of us are willing to extend a helping hand, but we're very reluctant to reach out for help when we need it ourselves. It's as if we've divided the world into 'those who offer help' and 'those who need help.' The truth is that we are both."*

In other words, accepting help is a part of giving help. As an advocate, you are giving of yourself daily; ensure that you are open to also receiving it.

BADASS DONATIONS MANAGER ACTIONS:

- ☐ You may not be comfortable asking for donations, but don't let your ego get in the way of much-needed support.

- ☐ First, understand the goal(s) of the monetary donation fund. Gain a clear idea of what the fund will pay for and what amount the patient and their family need to cover costs.

- ☐ Next, set up a simple way for donors to give money by creating an online fund for the patient.

- ☐ It is your duty to ethically manage the donation funds. If you aren't an immediate family member, work with the patient and their family to properly allocate the funds. The goal is to cover costs associated with the patient's illness and their basic needs.

- ☐ Anticipate ahead of time when funds will be needed. Then, don't hesitate to send tactful, gentle reminders to solicit donations.

- ☐ Eagerly accept non-monetary gifts. At the same time, be prepared to give suggestions when asked for ideas.

"Let food be thy medicine and medicine be thy food."

~ Hippocrates

The "Father of Medicine"

MEAL TRAIN ORGANIZER

Preparing and cooking meals may be the last thing the patient's family has the desire or strength to do. Suggesting a meal donation is always a good idea for people who are asking how they can help. If you live in a tight-knit community, you may not even need to ask. Either way, organizing the patient and their family's meals is a nice way to relieve some of their stress.

If you live with the patient, then asking others to donate meals to your household may be awkward. In that case, ask someone outside of your house to take on this role. Then, when asked by others for ways to support, you can direct them to the Meal Train Organizer.

MEAL TRAIN ORGANIZER'S RESPONSIBILITIES

The Meal Train Organizer will need to be someone who is well-organized. If people begin dropping off meals, someone will need to start organizing them. Organizing the meals prevents them from going to waste and being repetitive. Also, maybe you find there to be a lack of meals. Having someone solicit meal donations will help to supplement having to cook meals.

It also helps if the Meal Train Organizer is tech savvy. There are several digital meal train calendar options available. Whether it be through a website or an app, the Meal Train Organizer needs to create a calendar to stay organized. Plus, digital calendars help others to know when meals are needed.

The Meal Train Organizer may also need to take on tasks outside of organizing meals. For example, they may need to clean out the refrigerator or assist donors with the website. Also, if someone creates another meal train, they may want to combine them. This would eliminate confusion and an influx of meals.

MEAL TRAIN CALENDARS

Once the calendar is created, the Meal Train Organizer needs to share the link. Donors can then log on to the calendar to pick their date. Digital meal calendars are convenient because they allow donors to view available dates, see past meals, and sign up. For meal train service suggestions, head to www.badassadvocate.com/resources.

HOME DELIVERY MEAL KITS

Another way to make mealtime easier is to use home delivery meal kit services. There are multiple ways the Meal Train Organizer can handle the purchasing of meal kits. They can either create a home delivery meal kit fund or ask donators to purchase gift cards. Meal kits are delivered right to your front door, saving you time and energy.

Home delivery meal kits fall into one of two categories:

1. The company delivers a box that includes the ingredients and recipes. Someone will need to cook the meal. For most companies, preparing and cooking the meal takes an average of 30 minutes.

2. The meals arrive already prepared. All you need to do is heat them up.

Home delivery meal kit services are generally more expensive than shopping at the grocery. The benefit is they are convenient and can be useful in various situations:

1. For an entire family. The patient and their family can have the contents of a meal delivered. As mentioned, most meal kits require cooking. But the advantage of meal kits is that you don't have to go to the grocery or come up with an entire week's menu.

2. For those who are living in the same house as the sick loved one but don't want to eat the same meal as them. At times, the patient may prefer bland foods or have strict dietary needs. This can make meals unappealing for the healthy people in the house. Many meal kit companies pride themselves on healthy, tasty meals.

3. For the patient who has dietary restrictions. Some of these meal delivery services do cater to various diets, which can make it easier for the cook.

For a list of meal kit delivery companies and their offerings, go to www.badassadvocate.com/resources.

BADASS MEAL TRAIN ORGANIZER ACTIONS:

☐ Organize a meal train calendar for family and friends so meals aren't repeated or thrown away.

☐ Send communication explaining the meal train plan and how you will organize it.

☐ Speak to the patient about their and their family's dietary restrictions and food preferences. Be sure to share this information with donors.

☐ Take charge of all meal donation issues.

☐ Consider supplementing home-cooked meals with delivered meal kits. Meal kits can make mealtime quick and easy.

♡

"Power is gained by sharing knowledge, not hoarding it."

~ Unknown

VICE PRESIDENT OF COMMUNICATIONS

Dealing with someone you love being seriously ill can be emotionally and mentally exhausting. On top of that, you may have many well-intentioned people reaching out to offer their support. They may want to discuss the latest health updates or ask how they can help.

The thought of returning any form of communication can be overwhelming for those closely involved with the patient. Rehashing the details of the patient's illness can be a daunting task. If this is the case, I recommend creating the role of Vice President of Communications.

VP OF COMMUNICATIONS' RESPONSIBILITIES

If you want to add a VP of Communications, someone who is a clear communicator and tech savvy is a good fit. This person also needs to have enough decorum to know what should and should not be shared with a larger group. To take the burden off the caregivers, an extended family member or a good friend may be a good fit. Let me share with you how it can work.

> During my sister's illness, I lived halfway across the country. This meant I couldn't help with the day-to-day operations. The bulk of the responsibility fell on my family's shoulders. This was a harsh reality.

From the start, we received an influx of messages, phone calls, and questions about Meghan. I figured intercepting some of those would be a way I could help. This is when I gave myself the title of "VP of Communications." I figured if I was going to give myself a title it might as well be an elite one. Plus, it made my sister laugh, which was the entire point.

When Meghan was first diagnosed, my family made phone calls to extended family to let them know what was going on. We felt that hearing the bad news directly from us was the right thing to do. Plus, it gave us the opportunity to share our concerns, answer questions, and cry together.

Right around this time, I received a phone call from one of my cousins. He had a brother who had also dealt with a serious illness. He was calling to console me but also to give me some sage advice based on his experiences.

He presumed that since we were part of a big family, Meghan would likely hear from many who would want to help. He explained how those messages could be comforting but also overwhelming. His advice was that we not feel pressure to respond to every phone call, email, and text message we received. Instead, he urged me to take those messages as reminders that Meghan was loved, and that people were thinking of us.

He advised, "In fact, you may want to let people know that they shouldn't always expect a response. Putting this out there will alleviate pressure on you and your family."

I took his advice to heart. I didn't realize it at the time, but his advice would significantly reduce my family's stress in the months ahead.

Once a fair amount of our family and friends were aware of Meghan's illness, I decided it was time to step in. My thought was that I would take over the communication before it took over my family's lives. Before doing so, I gained their approval.

I explained that to relieve stress on them, I would take over sharing updates with family and friends. I insisted that they should not feel any pressure to reply to messages. Of course, they could respond if they wanted.

They agreed it was a good idea. They said the phone calls, text messages, and emails were very much appreciated. Hearing from so many people was touching. At the same time, they admitted they couldn't keep up. Even if replies weren't expected, my family felt obligated to respond. They were beginning to feel overwhelmed.

To keep it manageable, I set up three text message chains. One was for our dad's family, one was for our mom's family, and one was for Meghan's close friends. With such a large extended family, I would need certain relatives to represent their families. The plan was to ask them to pass the text on. Once they received my text, they would copy and paste it into a separate text message chain intended for their family.

For the friends' text message chain, I did the same. I asked them to pass the message on to Meghan's other good friends who would want updates.

In my first text message, I informed the recipients of the plan. I explained that I would be their main contact and that if they had questions and concerns about Meghan's health, they were more than welcome to contact me.

I also informed them that my intention wasn't to prevent them from contacting Meghan or my family. I encouraged them to continue sending cards, care packages, and text messages as they had been. My goal was to keep everyone informed while at the same time reducing correspondences. I warned everyone to not get their feelings hurt if messages to my family weren't returned.

After the initial message, I only sent a text when I had noteworthy news. I would type up a message with details of the update. I made sure to include the pertinent information but not divulge anything too private. Once I felt good about what was written, I would share it with Meghan for her approval.

This simple way of communicating to the masses worked great. In fact, one of Meghan's friends even mentioned the text chain at my sister's memorial. She explained how Meghan's long-distance friends liked being kept in the loop. The texts helped them to feel close to her. The texts signaled them when they needed to send love and support to Meghan.

A warning about sending mass communications via text is that it can be easily shared. Once the VP of Communications sends the text, they will have no control over who will read it. That means they need to be comfortable with people outside of the intended group reading it.

If they want to take it one step further, they can use a group communication app, such as Flock or Marco Polo. Group communication apps allow them to form group chats, share pictures, post videos, and so on. They also send alerts when a new message is posted. These apps are easy to set up.

Rally Cry

Another great benefit of the text chains was using them for a rally cry.

Imagine the impact on the psyche when a person goes from being a healthy adult to a frail and lethargic patient. It's rough, even for someone who is normally positive and happy. To watch someone you love in this kind of mental anguish is heart-wrenching. The group chat can be an easy way to communicate to others that the patient needs some extra love.

On days when Meghan seemed especially down, I would send out a mass text to summon the troops for their support. Boy, did these people deliver!

At the end of the day, I'd call her later to check in and see how she was feeling. It was clear her mood had changed. She would tell me all about the flurry of text messages she received throughout the day. Some were funny while others were sentimental. All were encouraging and appreciated.

I'm not quite sure if she knew the love messages were solicited, but that didn't matter. Her reaction was sweet either way. The important thing is that she knew that people were thinking of her and that she was loved. The power of positivity and love worked!

Conclusion

I don't want anyone to mistake what I am saying in this chapter. It's beautiful to have people reach out to your loved one! The issue isn't with their thoughtfulness. The challenge is that the patient and those closely involved are already in an arduous situation. So, feeling obligated to rehash details of the patient's case can be emotionally draining.

If you are in the beginning stages of informing people about the patient, be prepared for a bombardment of phone calls and messages. If this becomes too overwhelming, find a support team member to handle replies, preferably someone who isn't involved in the day-to-day caretaking. Managing these tasks gives a support team member a powerful way to contribute.

BADASS VP OF COMMUNICATIONS ACTIONS:

☐ Set up an easy way to communicate with close family and friends.

☐ Manage the communications string by sending regular messages with patient health updates.

☐ Be sure to gain approval from the patient, so you are clear on who to include in the text message chain.

☐ Prior to sending out the first message, work with the patient to decide on the information to be shared. Have the patient proofread the messages before hitting "send."

☐ In the first message, clearly explain the reasoning behind the text message chain. Transparency is always helpful.

☐ Have patience and grace when dealing with those who continually ask for updates. Understand their hearts are in a good place.

"Always leave people better than you found them. Hug the hurt. Kiss the broken. Befriend the lost. Love the lonely."

~ Unknown

DIRECTOR OF DELIGHT

Being seriously ill can cause a range of emotions, including fear, anger, and hopelessness. The Director of Delight is someone whose focus will be to lift the patient's spirits. A good fit for this role is someone who is naturally happy, fun, and creative.

DIRECTOR OF DELIGHT'S RESPONSIBILITIES

Besides comforting the patient, the Director of Delight can boost team members' attitudes. They can intentionally celebrate the army by organizing fun get-togethers. During this dark time, it's important for the group to set aside time to band together and pat one another on the back.

Cheering up others during a dark and difficult time can be challenging. I am not implying the Director of Delight can't have their own moments of sadness or frustration. Rather, they need to maintain a positive attitude around *the patient*. Since this can be a daunting task, it may be wise to assign more than one person to this role.

> During the summer of 2018, Meghan's health took a sharp turn for the worse. Around this time, I spoke to her about having visitors to help lift her spirits. She seemed depressed, which was hard to see, especially since that was out of character.

On top of not feeling great, she was seeing the same faces day in and day out which was not helping. It's important to understand that Meghan had always been a very social person. Now that she was stuck in the hospital, she was somewhat isolated. Illness, isolation, and a grim future were good reasons to be depressed.

Our family was also worn down. Keeping our spirits and energy up every day was a challenge. We too were scared and tired.

This is why I was surprised and thankful when Meghan announced she was up for visitors. To be clear, I'm referring to long-distance visitors. Meghan had several local friends who were wonderful and came to visit her often.

Immediately, Meghan and I began to create a list of who she'd like to come to visit. She had many friends and family members offering to come to Charleston to help. The goal was to invigorate, but not overwhelm, her.

After we organized a visitor schedule, I began making phone calls. The response was touching!

To our amazement, we quickly had a rotation of fresh-faced visitors. The new visitors also took on the exhausting job of staying overnight at the hospital. Meghan loved the sleepovers. She and the visitor would reminisce, laugh, and catch up on life. This was also a tremendous relief for our family.

If you haven't experienced this yet, sleeping in a hospital is quite the experience. You will most likely sleep on a partially-reclined chair or a hard couch. Throughout the night, you'll listen to a never-ending symphony of beeping machines. On top of that, you'll continually be awakened by middle-of-the-night vital sign checks. Needless to say, it is not a conducive environment for a good night's sleep.

The best part of this story is what happened *after* the visitors started to appear. We began to see a change in Meghan's emotional and mental state.

Right before this time, Meghan seemed down and very rarely smiled. After loved ones began to visit, she drastically changed. She started to smile and laugh again. Low and behold, her physical health began to change, too. She was getting stronger and more willing to start exercising again.

I cannot claim that 100% of her improvement was due to visitors. I can say that it was obvious they had a positive impact on Meghan's health. Even the nurses commented on her improvement since the visitor train arrived. They affirmed that they loved hearing the laughter coming from Meghan's room. They too saw a difference in her.

Several nurses commented that they felt laughter truly was the best medicine. They also advised that as long as we didn't have too many guests and they weren't too rowdy, they were happy for her to have visitors. They agreed that visitors were always a good thing for their patients. They wished that some patients had more.

More importantly, Meghan noticed a difference, too. She mentioned to me multiple times how happy and touched she was to have so many visitors.

Entertaining the Patient

Coming up with ideas of how to entertain someone who is bedridden or weak is not easy. I offer some suggestions below, but I encourage your team to brainstorm and come up with a list of their own. Also, make sure to check with the physician first before proceeding with any activity that may jeopardize the patient's health.

Old Photo Albums

Dig up some old photo albums and walk down memory lane. Reminiscing is a great opportunity to bring joy to the patient. Sharing some happy memories may even cause an eruption of belly laughing.

Portable Board Games

Patients can spend a lot of time sitting, so portable board games may be a good choice. Games like Travel Scrabble®, Battleship®, and Scattergories® can be a lot of fun. Cards are also a great choice because there are endless possibilities of games to play.

Last, although they are a lot of fun, be sensitive to whether the patient is up for games that tend to be loud. Games like Yahtzee™ or Boggle® may be disturbing.

Mind-Sharpening Activities

Mind-sharpening activities, like crossword puzzles, can also be pleasurable. Not only are they quiet activities that the patient can do on their own, but they may bestow some added benefits. Research has shown that people who engage in "puzzle" games have better memory and cognitive skills.[15] Encouraging the patient to routinely work on word puzzles could help improve their brain functioning.

Some other activities patients may enjoy are adult coloring books, Sudoku, and jigsaw puzzles. If the patient enjoys jigsaw puzzles, I would recommend buying a puzzle mat. The mat can help you to easily roll up the puzzle and put it away when not needed.

BODY TREATMENTS

A great way to spoil the patient is to treat them to a massage, pedicure, or manicure. Please check with the physician first to ensure it is safe for them to receive body treatments. If approved and the patient is homebound, consider hiring someone to come to the house. During hospital stays, you may want to ask the nurse or palliative care provider if they offer these services.

If having a professional come to the house isn't an option, the Director of Delight can consider doing it themselves. My sister's daughters gave her a few pedicures while she was sick. Not only were the pedicures relaxing, but they also were a great way for them to bond. If pedicures are something the patient loves, buy a foot bath and recreate the feeling of going to the spa.

EDIBLE TREATS

If the patient has strict dietary needs, a special treat may be challenging to find. However, many food companies cater to specific diets these days. Head to www.badassadvocate.com/resources to find a list of ideas. Also, you may want to check out local businesses to save on shipping costs.

---

[15] www.exeter.ac.uk/news/featurednews/title_595009_en.html

CONCLUSION

As the Director of Delight, once you come up with a list of fun ideas, create a plan of action. You are more likely to execute on them if there is a plan in place. Following through will be an important aspect of this role. Having great ideas written down won't bring the patient joy but acting on them will.

Pay close attention to the patient's behavior and mood. The Director of Delight will want to choose activities based on the patient's mood that day. One day the patient may feel great and be up for something new while the next day they may feel lousy and prefer to rest. Be prepared to bend to their needs. The Director of Delight should do their best to not get disappointed if their plan doesn't work out exactly as they imagined.

The Director of Delight has an important role. Having someone own the role of bringing joy to the patient may have more of an impact on the patient than you think.

BADASS DIRECTOR OF DELIGHT ACTIONS:

☐ Think of creative ways to bring the patient joy within the confines of their abilities.

☐ Make a list of activities that will satisfy the patient's needs & preferences.

☐ Speak to the patient's physician about the activities you are planning. The point is to ensure any activity will not jeopardize the patient's health and progression.

☐ Be aware of when the patient doesn't feel well and understand their limitations.

☐ Remember not everything needs to have grandeur. The goal is to lift the patient's spirits. Little gestures can bring just as much joy as the big ones.

☐ Aim to bring happiness when you can, staying consistent during the roller coaster ride of good and bad days.

Acknowledgments

To **Meghan and Dad**, I miss you both every day. Thank you for setting amazing life examples. In so many ways, you taught me what it means to be kind, loving, and patient. I would give anything to bring you back. Since that isn't possible, at the very least, I hope the lessons we learned from your illnesses will help others. I know both of you would want the same.

To my husband, **Kevin**, who tolerated my constant writing and distracted mind. You were my rock during Meghan's illness, and I wouldn't have been the advocate I was if it wasn't for your support. I couldn't have completed this book without you. I love you with all my heart.

To my sweet boy, **Graham**. Having you next to me every morning while I wrote will be a memory I'll cherish. My favorite part was when you would randomly reach over and touch my arm with your little hand. You motivate me every day to set a good example and accomplish big things in life. I love your spunk, funny facial expressions, and outgoing personality. Your kind soul makes my heart swell, and I'm so thankful you made me a mom.

To my beautiful daughter, **Mallory**. I am the luckiest stepmom in the world to have you as my daughter. You are kind, thoughtful, and fun. Thank you for cheering me on throughout this entire journey of writing and for believing in me. When you told me that one day I'd "be on the New York Times Best Sellers List," it built my confidence. Thank you for being such a wonderful person.

To my sweet nieces, **Haley & Hannah**. Some day when you become mothers yourself, you will realize how much your mom loved you. She is a part of you, and I see her wonderful attributes in both of you every time I'm with you. She was blessed to have you, and you are lucky to be born her daughters. For the rest of my life, I will be here to help your hearts heal.

To my **Mom**. You've endured so much, and I'm sorry life didn't give you more breaks. You taught all of us what it takes to be a great caretaker. You constantly sacrificed and gave yourself to both Dad and Meghan. Without you, this book wouldn't be possible. Thank you for everything you've ever done for me. Your input and memory for this book were invaluable. Thank you for your unwavering love and support.

To my brother, **Michael**. Your encouragement to write this book motivated me to keep going when the writing got tough. As Meghan's other sibling, I know her death has been equally as heartbreaking for you. She was your partner in crime since age 1½. You were her rock when she was sick. I know she was so thankful for all the support you gave her and her family.

To my brother-in-law, **Greg**. Words cannot express how sorry I am that you had to lose your sweet wife. I know how much you loved her and that your heart hurts, especially for your girls. I will always be here to help your little family get through the pain.

To my sisters-in-law, **Page** and **Tanya**. We may not be sisters by blood, but I love you both so much. Thank you for always cheering me on and supporting me while I was writing.

To my dear friends, **Kelly** and **Mary**. If it wasn't for the two of you, I wouldn't have survived this heartbreaking time. Thank you for always having my back, loving me unconditionally, and letting me talk your ear off without judgment. We aren't sisters by birth but by choice.

To **Aunt Mary, Aunt Re, Colleen, Jenny H, Joanne, Julie, Katie, Kirsten, Missy,** and **Robin**. For many months after Meghan's passing you consistently checked on me to see how I was doing. A simple "thank you" doesn't seem like enough. After someone dies, the world must move on, and for those who are grieving deeply, it's a harsh reality. Thank you for taking the time to reach out to me and remind me I wasn't alone.

To **Dr. Aron**. Words could never express my gratitude towards you. First, you took amazing care of my sister and helped to give her peace during a most vulnerable time. You have a gift for making the severely sick feel comfortable and supported. Second, not only did you write a beautiful foreword, but you gave me invaluable advice during my writing process. Your kindness, generosity, and authenticity are what make you an amazing human being. Because of these attributes, every patient and family member that comes into contact with you is blessed.

To **Amanda Fowler**. First, thank you for the care you gave Meghan. You and the rest of the oncology team held a special place in Meghan's heart. Second, thank you for reading this book in its rawest form and for giving me feedback. Every time I asked your expert opinion, you were happy to give me your thoughts. Hearing what you thought was so helpful.

To the rest of my thoughtful family members, friends, and co-workers. I'm sorry if I didn't mention you by name, but it is not possible. This book would have taken me twice as long to write.

There were so many of you who gave warm hugs, wrote sweet notes, and sent generous donations. I cannot thank you enough for your continual kindness and love. We couldn't have survived those challenging times without you.

We know that you adored Meghan and Dad like we did. They appreciated everything you did for them, and it warms our hearts to know they were beloved.

About the Author

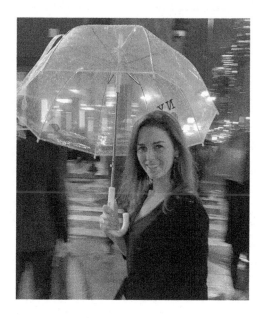

Erin Mulqueen Galyean is a professional author and public speaker who trains sales professionals in effective communication with healthcare providers. She lost her father to Non-Hodgkin's Lymphoma in 1997 and her sister to a rare lung disease in 2018. Fueled by these heartbreaking personal experiences, Erin decided her vision is to help others powerfully advocate for the seriously ill loved one in their life.

♡

Thank You!

Dear Reader, I would greatly appreciate it if you'd leave an honest review of my book. Not only will it help others to determine if this is the right book for them, but it helps me to learn as well. My goal is to help others who are in a similar situation get through this challenging time.

Most of all, I hope reading this book was helpful for you and gave you a new perspective on advocating. If you would like additional support or ideas, please visit www.badassadvocate.com.

Made in the USA
Monee, IL
22 December 2020